Bee Healthy Diabetic Log Book

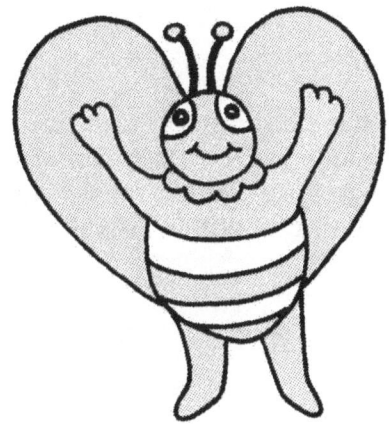

Sharon B. Barker

iUniverse, Inc.

New York Lincoln Shanghai

Bee Healthy Diabetic Log Book

iUniverse, Inc.

For information address:
iUniverse
2021 Pine Lake Road, Suite 100
Lincoln, NE 68512
www.iuniverse.com

Remember to consult your doctor before making any changes to your dietary or medicinal plan.

ISBN: 0-595-27117-0

Printed in the United States of America

Bee Healthy Diabetic Log Book

This Log Book belongs to:

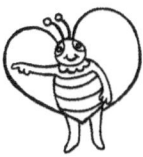

Name: _____

Address: _____

_____

Phone: _____

In case of emergency, call: _____
I have type 1 or type 2 (circle one) diabetes.
The current medicine(s) I take are: _____

_____

_____

Important Numbers

My clinic/physician's phone number: _____

My pharmacist's phone number: _____

My dentist's phone number: _____

My eye doctor's phone number: _____

My diabetes educator's phone number: _____

My dietitian's phone number: _____

The "*Bee* Healthy" Log Book was inspired by my desire to bring sunshine to people who have been recently diagnosed with diabetes, or who have lived with diabetes for years. I was diagnosed in 2001 with type II diabetes, at the age of thirty-one. I know first hand the day to day, and sometimes, hour to hour challenges that come with diabetes. I had to learn how to eat differently, exercise more often, take medicine regularly and record my own blood readings. It wasn't easy at times, yet each day I learned more about my body and how to stay healthy. For us, taking glucose readings should be part of the everyday routine. Diabetics need to incorporate this healthy habit into their life right away. This helps you and your doctor see a pattern in your body's ability to utilize glucose.

It's also a good idea to journal how you feel, both physically and emotionally. Diabetes can evoke a wide range of feelings, including frustration, sadness, anger, helplessness and fear. I've known all of these, as well as the triumph of getting diabetes under control. Yet, many times I wonder if my adjustment to diabetes would have been faster if someone had encouraged me to see a positive side. A positive side to diabetes, you ask? Well, why not?

In your hands is my ideal log book, with a positive side. It is designed to make logging your daily glucose readings and journaling how you feel simple, and, hopefully, uplifting. It is filled with reminders to love and care for yourself, encouraging you to see your diabetes care as one aspect of your master plan for well-being. It also comes with an optional chart to trend your weekly readings. Why did I choose bees for inspiration? A bee's life centers on making honey (sugar), not too different from our ever present goal of managing it. My hope is that these charming, light hearted bees help you smile both on sunny and cloudy days. May this disease never crush your dreams or change how you see yourself. Remember, you define yourself, not diabetes. Always *bee*lieve in yourself!

I dedicate this book to my husband, Jai, my soul mate and best friend. He has always *bee*lieved in me. He even tested his blood the first time, when I was too scared to test myself, to show me how easy it is to test. Thanks, Jai, for the long hours editing this book, I love you so much! I also dedicate this book to my five *bee*autiful cats and their unconditional love, and to my Dad, who's advice on living with diabetes has been priceless. Special thanks to my Diabetes Educator, Margie Goebel, R.N. (C.D.E.), who was so gentle the day I was diagnosed and gave such insightful diabetes classes. Finally, but most importantly, I dedicate this log book to all the "bees" in the world that bravely live with diabetes every day.

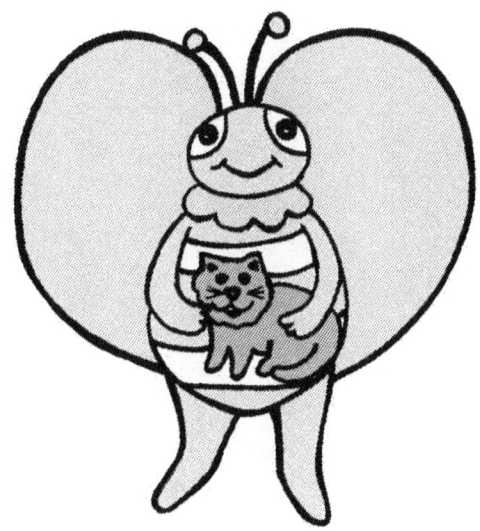

The following charts are intended for informational purposes only and cannot serve for the care provided by a licensed physician. Seek medical guidance before making any changes to your individual health care program.

The American Diabetes Association's recommendation for glycemic control for non-pregnant individuals with diabetes

Whole Blood Values	Glucose (mg/dl)
Average before meal goal	80 to 120
Bedtime goal	100 to 140
HbA1C (%) Test every three months at a medical facility	Below 7

Note: Patients with co morbid diseases, the very young and older adults, and others with unusual conditions or circumstances may warrant different treatment goals.

Your doctor's recommendation for your blood glucose goals

Glucose Reading (mg/dl)

Before meal target range   _____

After meal target range   _____

Dietitian's carbohydrate recommendation per day _____

Quarterly HbA1c(%) target goal   _____

Other Test Results

Your HbA1c(%) Test Results

Date: _____ Date: _____ Date: _____
Date: _____ Date: _____ Date: _____

Your Cholesterol Test Results

Date: _____ Date: _____ Date: _____
Date: _____ Date: _____ Date: _____

Weight Recordings

Date: _____ Date: _____ Date: _____
Date: _____ Date: _____ Date: _____
Date: _____ Date: _____ Date: _____
Date: _____ Date: _____ Date: _____

Blood Pressure Recordings

Date: _____ Date: _____ Date: _____
Date: _____ Date: _____ Date: _____
Date: _____ Date: _____ Date: _____
Date: _____ Date: _____ Date: _____

Eye Exams

Date: _____ Date: _____ Date: _____

Dental Exams

Date: _____ Date: _____ Date: _____

Foot Exams

Date: _____ Date: _____ Date: _____

Carbohydrate Conversion Chart

If you have chosen to use Carbohydrate Choices to manage your blood sugar level, the chart below will help you make your conversions.

Carbohydrate Conversion Chart	
Total Carbohydrate Grams	**Carbohydrate Choices**
0-5	0
6-10	½
11-20	1
21-25	1½
26-35	2
36-40	2½
41-50	3
51-55	3½
56-65	4
66-70	4½
71-80	5

From *My Food Plan,* © 2000 International Diabetes Center, Minneapolis, USA.
Used with permission.

"Fifteen grams of carbohydrate equal one Carbohydrate Choice."

Carbohydrate Food Charts

Use this chart to determine the amount of carbohydrate in a typical serving of food. Since carbohydrate amounts vary slightly between products and brands of food, below are the averages of several types. We encourage you to use these for educational purposes, but not as a substitute for the advice of your physician or dietician. You will want to read food labels and choose low-fat, low-salt, healthy foods. Remember to plan your meals and spread your carbohydrate consumption out throughout the day. Don't skip meals! Consult your physician or dietician for advice on your individual food plan.

"Approximately 15 grams of carbohydrate equal one Carbohydrate Choice."

Fruits and Vegetables	Serving Size	Carbohydrate grams
Apple	1 medium	15
Banana	1 medium	30
Beans, baked	½ cup	22
Beans, garbanzo, kidney and pinto	½ cup	15
Blueberries	1 cup	15
Cantaloupe	1 cup in cubes	15
Corn	½ cup	15
French fries	4 oz	25
Fruit, dried	½ cup	30
Fruit juice, apple	1 cup	30
Fruit juice, grape	1 cup	40
Fruit juice, orange juice	1 cup	25
Grapefruit	½ medium	15
Honeydew	1 cup in cubes	15
Orange	1 medium	15
Pear	1 medium	15
Peas, green	½ cup	15
Potato, baked or boiled	1 small (3 oz)	16
Potato, baked or boiled	1 large (8 oz)	40
Potato, mashed with milk/margarine	1 cup	31
Prunes	3 prunes	15
Raisins	2 tablespoons	15
Raspberries	1 cup	15
Squash, cooked	1 cup	15
Strawberries	1 cup	15
Vegetables, cooked	1 cup	10
Vegetables, raw	1 cup	5
Watermelon	1 cup in cubes	15

Breads, Grains and Beans	Serving Size	Carbohydrate grams
Bagel, plain white or multigrain	3 oz	45-55
Bagel, raison	3 oz	60
Biscuit	2 x 2 inches	11
Breadcrumbs	1 tablespoon	7
Bread, French	1 slice	23
Bread, seven grain	1 slice	19
Bread, wheat or white	1 thin slice	15
Bread, wheat or white	1 thick slice	20
Bread, pita pocket	2 oz	32
Bun, hamburger	3 oz	45
Cereal, cold and ready-to-eat	pkg. serving	18-26
Cereal, cooked (oatmeal)	½ cup	15
Croissant	2 x 2 inches	30
Croutons	1 oz	12-17
Dinner roll, soft	small	15
Muffin, English	2 oz	30
Pancakes,	2 pancakes, 4" across	15
Pasta, cooked (macaroni, noodles, spaghetti)	1 cup	30
Rice, white, short/med grain, hot/cooked	1 cup	54
Rice, brown, short/med grain, hot/cooked	1 cup	46
Rice, wild, cooked	1 cup	35
Stuffing, prepared and cooked	1 cup	22
Taco shell	1 small	6-8
Tortilla	1 tortilla, 12" across	30
Waffle	1 waffle, 8" across	30

Milk, Yogurt and Milk Substitutes	Serving Size	Carbohydrate grams
Cheese, low fat cottage	½ cup	3
Cheese, American, Swiss	1 slice	1
Milk, skim, 1% or 2%	1 cup	12
Milk, chocolate	1 cup	26
Rice, beverage	½-3/4 cup (4-6 oz)	15-17
Soy milk, low-fat or nonfat, plain	1 cup (8oz)	15
Yogurt, low-fat, all flavors	6 oz	23-28
Yogurt, with fruit	1 cup (8 oz)	43

Combination Foods	Serving Size	Carbohydrate grams
Chicken Chow Mein (includes rice)	pkg. serving	53
Burrito, bean	½ - 2 cups	53
Burrito, beef	1½ - 2 cups	38
Frozen dinner	1 dinner, 8-11oz	31-46
Gravies, sauces & dips	¼ cup	1-8
Macaroni and cheese	pkg. serving	44
Pizza, thick-crust, medium	1 slice (1/8 pizza)	33-45
Pizza, thin-crust, pepperoni	1 slice (1/8 pizza)	22
Soup, beef, bean, noodle or vegetable	1 cup	8-15
Soup, chicken broth	1 cup	1
Soup, chicken noodle	1 cup	9
Soup, cream of mushroom	½ cup, condensed	9
Soup, New England clam chowder	1 cup	16
Soup, split pea & ham	1 cup	29
Soup, tomato	1 cup	17
Spaghetti sauce	½ cup	10
Sub sandwich	1 sub, 6" long	34-49

Snacks & Desserts	Serving Size	Carbohydrate grams
Brownie (no frosting)	3 oz	47
Cake, cheese	3 oz	25
Cake, plain angel food	2 oz	24
Cakes, rice (most flavors)	1 cake	9-15
Chips, potato, corn or tortilla	10-15 chips (1oz)	15-17
Chocolate bar (with nuts)	2 oz	30
Cookie, chocolate chip	1 oz.	15
Crackers, graham	1 square, 2 ½ inches	5
Crackers, saltines	2 crackers	5
Donut (no frosting)	1 donut	25
Ice cream, vanilla	½ cup	16-23
Jell-O, all flavors	½ cup	19
Jell-O, sugar free	½ cup	0
Muffin (no frosting)	1 oz	13
Syrup, diet pancake	¼ cup	12
Pie, apple, cherry, blueberry	1/8 of 9" pie	47
Pie, pumpkin	1/8 of 9" pie	29
Popcorn, unbuttered	3 cups	15
Pretzels, hard	1 oz	20-23
Pudding, all flavors	4 oz	28

Low Carbohydrate Foods & Drinks	Serving Size	Carbohydrate grams
Catsup/Mustard	1 tablespoon	4/5
Cheese, string, low-fat	1 oz (1 stick)	1
Coffee/Tea, without sugar	unlimited	0
Egg, cooked or raw	1 egg	0
Fruit flavored drinks with sugar substitutes	1 cup	0
Gelatin (diet)	½ cup	0
Herbs, fresh - like cilantro and oregano, these are great flavor enhancers!		0
Jellies, sugar free	1 teaspoon	5
Mayonnaise	1 tablespoon	1
Meat, pork/chicken/beef (7 grams of fat or less)	3 oz.	4-6
Pickle, dill	1 large	3
Salad dressings, low fat or fat free	2 tablespoons	2-6
Salsa	2 tablespoons	4
Soda, diet with sugar substitutes	unlimited	0
Spices – check for salt!	unlimited	0
Sugar, honey	1 teaspoon	4-5
Sugar substitute	1 packet	1
Tofu	1/5 pound	1
Water – It's natural and great for your body!	unlimited	0

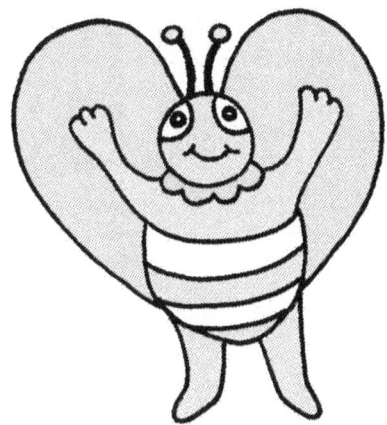

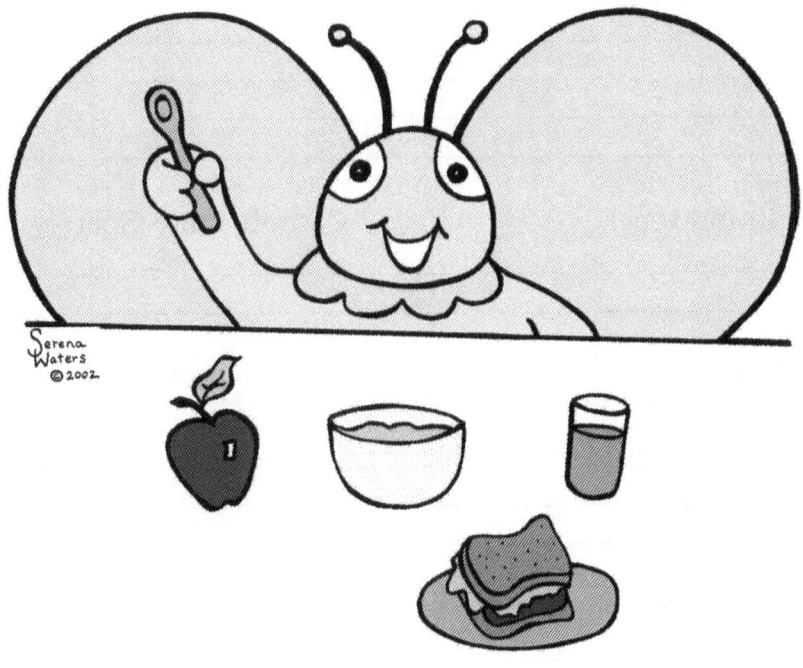

Beeing healthy means eating healthy!

My Meal Plan

Breakfast   Carbohydrate Goal _____

_____
_____
_____
_____

Midmorning snack   Carbohydrate Goal _____

_____
_____

Lunchtime   Carbohydrate Goal _____

_____
_____
_____
_____

Afternoon Snack   Carbohydrate Goal _____

_____
_____

Supper   Carbohydrate Goal _____

_____
_____
_____
_____

Bedtime Snack   Carbohydrate Goal _____

_____
_____

Total Carbohydrates _____

Body Signs
Listen to your body, it's telling you something.

The following signs may be telling you that you might be experiencing high or low blood sugar levels. If you experience any of these or other symptoms, please consult your physician. Don't be afraid to call for assistance if you sense you might not be able to help yourself out of a situation.

Test your blood often to assess whether your blood glucose level is normal, high or low. Take your medicine/insulin as instructed by your doctor or pharmacist.

Symptoms of High Blood Sugar

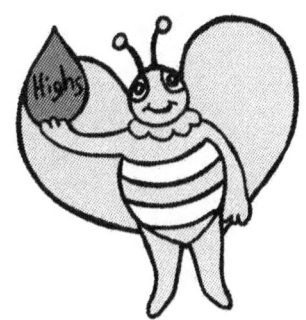

Extra thirsty
Extra hungry, cravings for sugar/carbohydrates
Extra tired
Frequent urination
Blurry vision
Lack of energy
Dry, itchy skin
Weak legs
Dizziness
Question: Do you have a cold, did you skip a meal or eat too many carbohydrates? Is your medicine or insulin right for you?

Symptoms of Low Blood Sugar

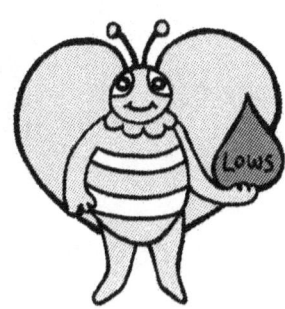

Feeling shaky, sweaty
Irritable or angry
Anxiousness
Numbness
Tingling in lips or elsewhere
Inability to think clearly
Dizziness, weak legs
Loud noises and bright lights are irritating
Clumsy, dropping things
Questions: Did you skip a meal or were you exercising? Is your medicine or insulin right for you?

Author's note: I keep small, healthy snacks with me at all times to help prevent blood sugar lows.

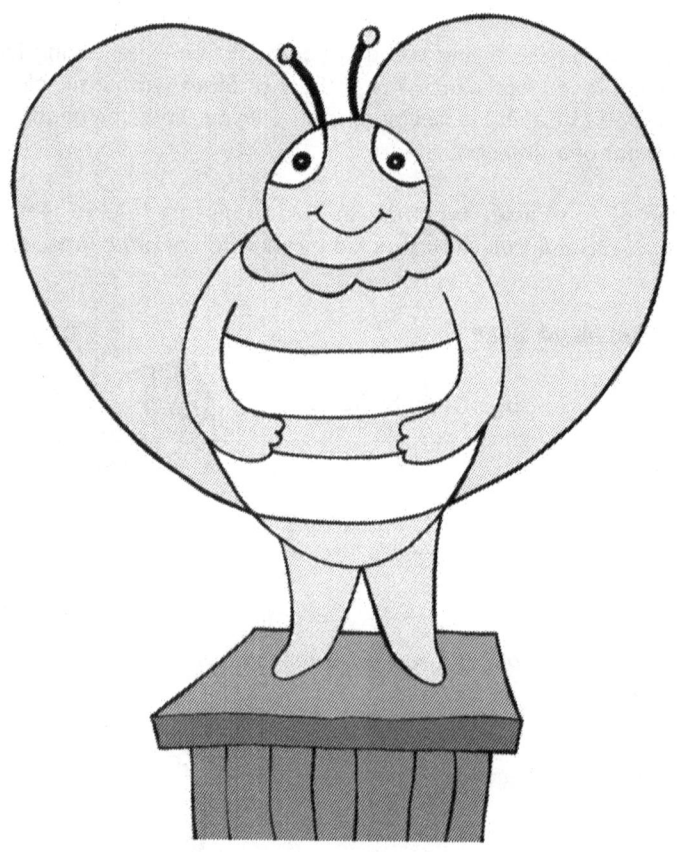

Put yourself on a pedestal. You're important!

Stress Busters
Stress can affect glucose. Here are some ideas to lower stress:

Out and About

Spend some time in nature, walking or hiking
Exercise / do some gentle stretches
Volunteer with an organization of your choice; giving feels good
Get a massage at a spa or health facility
Have your hair done at a salon, and ask them to massage your scalp
Meditate in a quiet place or visit a spiritual center
Listen to your favorite music, sing or dance with friends
Go shopping for something you can afford
Take a vacation from work to a relaxing destination
Take a "Sunday" drive, or go for a bike ride
Watch or play your favorite sport
Take up outdoor photography
Go to the ocean or a lake
Go to an amusement park
Plant flowers or a garden

At Home

Write your feelings in a journal
Take a nap to energize yourself
Paint or draw a picture
Think of a happy moment in your life
Play a board game or cards
Take a relaxing bubble bath
Give a hug to yourself or somebody else
Work on your favorite hobby or pastime
Spend time with a loved one or a pet
Read a good book or magazine
Watch no news for one day, or watch something positive
Do some woodworking
Call to chat with a "positive minded" friend or relative
Drink a glass of water to hydrate your body
Watch your favorite television show or a funny movie to make you laugh
Work on photo albums, write a letter, sew or cook a new recipe
Breathe deeply and concentrate on your breath until you feel relaxed

Here's how you can you use your daily journal.

Time	Monday, March 13th Meals and snacks	Carbs or Exchanges	Glucose Reading Pre	Glucose Reading Post	Insulin	Meds
8am	1 small muffin ½ cup orange juice 1 cup yogurt (20g. carbs)	3	140 8am	169 10am		1 actos 2 amaryl
Noon	(Tuna Sandwich) 2 slices of bread 1 medium banana	4	120 noon	163 2pm		
3pm	3 cups Popcorn	1	134 3pm			
5pm	2 slices thin crust pizza 1½ cup green salad 1 T. fat free dressing	3	95 5pm	151 8pm		1 amaryl
9pm	1 cup Strawberry jello	2	140 9pm			

Carbohydrates / Exchanges __13__ Total __13-14__ Goal

Journal your exercise, thoughts or feelings here.   Ketones _____

Felt dizzy after supper, but I went for a 1 hour walk and felt better. ✳ Get refills tomorrow.

Time	Monday,_____ Meals and snacks	Carbs or Exchanges	Glucose Reading		Insulin	Meds
			Pre	Post		

Carbohydrates / Exchanges _____ Total _____ Goal

Journal your exercise, thoughts or feelings here.   Ketones _____

_____

_____

_____

Time	Tuesday,_____ Meals and snacks	Carbs or Exchanges	Glucose Reading		Insulin	Meds
			Pre	Post		

Carbohydrates / Exchanges _____ **Total** _____ **Goal**

Journal your exercise, thoughts or feelings here.   Ketones _____

_____

_____

_____

Time	Wednesday,_____ Meals and snacks	Carbs or Exchanges	Glucose Reading		Insulin	Meds
			Pre	Post		

Carbohydrates / Exchanges _____ **Total** _____ **Goal**

Journal your exercise, thoughts or feelings here.   Ketones _____

_____

_____

_____

Time	Thursday,_____ Meals and snacks	Carbs or Exchanges	Glucose Reading		Insulin	Meds
			Pre	Post		

Carbohydrates / Exchanges _____ **Total** _____ **Goal**

Journal your exercise, thoughts or feelings here.   Ketones _____

_____

_____

_____

Time	Friday,_____ Meals and snacks	Carbs or Exchanges	Glucose Reading		Insulin	Meds
			Pre	Post		

Carbohydrates / Exchanges _____ **Total** _____ **Goal**

Journal your exercise, thoughts or feelings here.   Ketones _____

_____

_____

_____

Time	Saturday,_____ Meals and snacks	Carbs or Exchanges	Glucose Reading Pre	Glucose Reading Post	Insulin	Meds

Carbohydrates / Exchanges _____ **Total** _____ **Goal**

Journal your exercise, thoughts or feelings here.   Ketones _____

_____
_____
_____

Time	Sunday,_____ Meals and snacks	Carbs or Exchanges	Glucose Reading		Insulin	Meds
			Pre	Post		

Carbohydrates / Exchanges _____ Total _____ Goal

Journal your exercise, thoughts or feelings here.   Ketones _____

_____

_____

_____

Week of _____

Blood Glucose Summary

Time	Mon		Tues		Wed		Thurs		Fri		Sat		Sun	
	Pre	Post	Pre	Post	Pre	Post	Pre	Post	Pre	Post	Pre	Post	Pre	Post
Average														

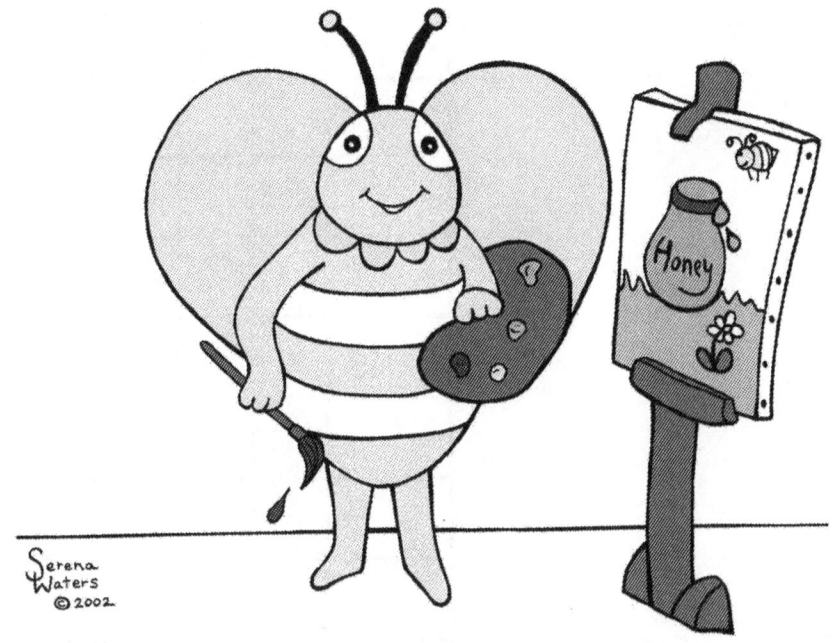

Bee creative! You are the artist of your life. Paint away!

Time	Monday,_____ Meals and snacks	Carbs or Exchanges	Glucose Reading		Insulin	Meds
			Pre	Post		
Carbohydrates / Exchanges _____ **Total** _____ **Goal**						

Journal your exercise, thoughts or feelings here.   Ketones _____

_____

_____

_____

Time	Tuesday,_____ Meals and snacks	Carbs or Exchanges	Glucose Reading		Insulin	Meds
			Pre	Post		

Carbohydrates / Exchanges _____ Total _____ Goal

Journal your exercise, thoughts or feelings here.   Ketones _____

_____
_____
_____

Time	Wednesday,_____ Meals and snacks	Carbs or Exchanges	Glucose Reading		Insulin	Meds
			Pre	Post		

Carbohydrates / Exchanges _____ **Total** _____ **Goal**

Journal your exercise, thoughts or feelings here.   Ketones _____

_____

_____

_____

Time	Thursday,_____ Meals and snacks	Carbs or Exchanges	Glucose Reading		Insulin	Meds
			Pre	Post		

Carbohydrates / Exchanges _____ **Total** _____ **Goal**

Journal your exercise, thoughts or feelings here.   Ketones _____

_____

_____

_____

Time	Friday,_____ Meals and snacks	Carbs or Exchanges	Glucose Reading Pre	Post	Insulin	Meds

Carbohydrates / Exchanges _____ **Total** _____ **Goal**

Journal your exercise, thoughts or feelings here.   Ketones _____

_____
_____
_____

Time	Saturday,_____ Meals and snacks	Carbs or Exchanges	Glucose Reading		Insulin	Meds
			Pre	Post		

Carbohydrates / Exchanges _____ **Total** _____ **Goal**

Journal your exercise, thoughts or feelings here.   Ketones _____

_____
_____
_____

Time	Sunday,_____ Meals and snacks	Carbs or Exchanges	Glucose Reading		Insulin	Meds
			Pre	Post		

Carbohydrates / Exchanges _____ Total _____ Goal

Journal your exercise, thoughts or feelings here.   Ketones _____

_____

_____

_____

Week of _____

Blood Glucose Summary

Time	Mon		Tues		Wed		Thurs		Fri		Sat		Sun	
	Pre	Post	Pre	Post	Pre	Post	Pre	Post	Pre	Post	Pre	Post	Pre	Post
Average														

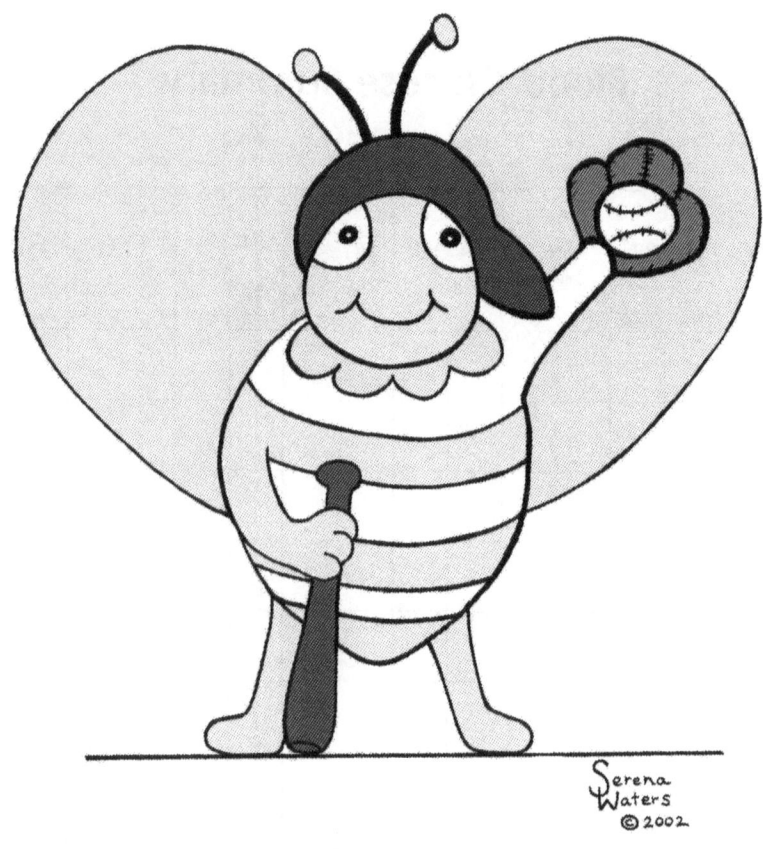

Bee playful! Catch the spirit! You are young at heart!

Time	Monday,_____ Meals and snacks	Carbs or Exchanges	Glucose Reading		Insulin	Meds
			Pre	Post		

Carbohydrates / Exchanges _____ Total _____ Goal

Journal your exercise, thoughts or feelings here.   Ketones _____

_____

_____

_____

Time	Tuesday,_____ Meals and snacks	Carbs or Exchanges	Glucose Reading		Insulin	Meds
			Pre	Post		

Carbohydrates / Exchanges _____ **Total** _____ **Goal**

Journal your exercise, thoughts or feelings here.   Ketones _____

_____
_____
_____

Time	Wednesday,_____ Meals and snacks	Carbs or Exchanges	Glucose Reading		Insulin	Meds
			Pre	Post		

Carbohydrates / Exchanges _____ **Total** _____ **Goal**

Journal your exercise, thoughts or feelings here.   Ketones _____

_____

_____

_____

Time	Thursday,_____ Meals and snacks	Carbs or Exchanges	Glucose Reading		Insulin	Meds
			Pre	Post		

Carbohydrates / Exchanges _____ **Total** _____ **Goal**

Journal your exercise, thoughts or feelings here.   Ketones _____

_____

_____

_____

Time	Friday,_____ Meals and snacks	Carbs or Exchanges	Glucose Reading Pre	Post	Insulin	Meds
Carbohydrates / Exchanges _____ **Total** _____ **Goal**						

Journal your exercise, thoughts or feelings here.   Ketones _____

_____
_____
_____

Time	Saturday,_____ Meals and snacks	Carbs or Exchanges	Glucose Reading		Insulin	Meds
			Pre	Post		

Carbohydrates / Exchanges _____ **Total** _____ **Goal**

Journal your exercise, thoughts or feelings here.   Ketones _____

_____

_____

_____

Time	Sunday,_____ Meals and snacks	Carbs or Exchanges	Glucose Reading		Insulin	Meds
			Pre	Post		

Carbohydrates / Exchanges _____ **Total** _____ **Goal**

Journal your exercise, thoughts or feelings here.   Ketones _____

_____
_____
_____

Week of _____

Blood Glucose Summary

Time	Mon		Tues		Wed		Thurs		Fri		Sat		Sun	
	Pre	Post	Pre	Post	Pre	Post	Pre	Post	Pre	Post	Pre	Post	Pre	Post
Average														

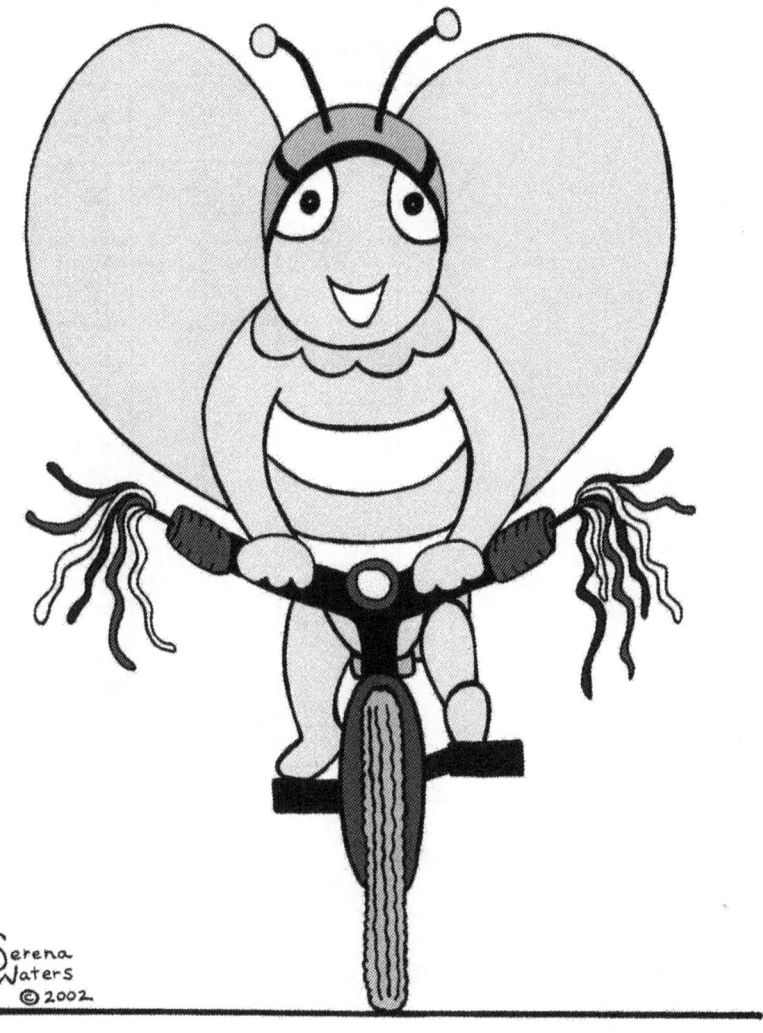

Bee confident! You'll be great. Courage is inside you.

Time	Monday,_____ Meals and snacks	Carbs or Exchanges	Glucose Reading		Insulin	Meds
			Pre	Post		

Carbohydrates / Exchanges _____ Total _____ Goal

Journal your exercise, thoughts or feelings here.   Ketones _____

_____

_____

_____

Time	Tuesday,_____ Meals and snacks	Carbs or Exchanges	Glucose Reading		Insulin	Meds
			Pre	Post		
Carbohydrates / Exchanges _____ **Total** _____ **Goal**						

Journal your exercise, thoughts or feelings here.   Ketones _____

_____
_____
_____

Time	Wednesday,_____ Meals and snacks	Carbs or Exchanges	Glucose Reading		Insulin	Meds
			Pre	Post		

Carbohydrates / Exchanges _____ Total _____ Goal

Journal your exercise, thoughts or feelings here.   Ketones _____

_____

_____

_____

Time	Thursday,_____ Meals and snacks	Carbs or Exchanges	Glucose Reading		Insulin	Meds
			Pre	Post		

Carbohydrates / Exchanges _____ **Total** _____ **Goal**

Journal your exercise, thoughts or feelings here.   Ketones _____

_____
_____
_____

Time	Friday,_____ Meals and snacks	Carbs or Exchanges	Glucose Reading		Insulin	Meds
			Pre	Post		

Carbohydrates / Exchanges _____ **Total** _____ **Goal**

Journal your exercise, thoughts or feelings here.   Ketones _____

_____
_____
_____

Time	Saturday,_____ Meals and snacks	Carbs or Exchanges	Glucose Reading		Insulin	Meds
			Pre	Post		
Carbohydrates / Exchanges _____ **Total** _____ **Goal**						

Journal your exercise, thoughts or feelings here.   Ketones _____

_____

_____

_____

Time	Sunday,_____ Meals and snacks	Carbs or Exchanges	Glucose Reading		Insulin	Meds
			Pre	Post		

Carbohydrates / Exchanges _____ **Total** _____ **Goal**

Journal your exercise, thoughts or feelings here.   Ketones _____

_____

_____

_____

Week of _____

Blood Glucose Summary

Time	Mon		Tues		Wed		Thurs		Fri		Sat		Sun	
	Pre	Post	Pre	Post	Pre	Post	Pre	Post	Pre	Post	Pre	Post	Pre	Post
Average														

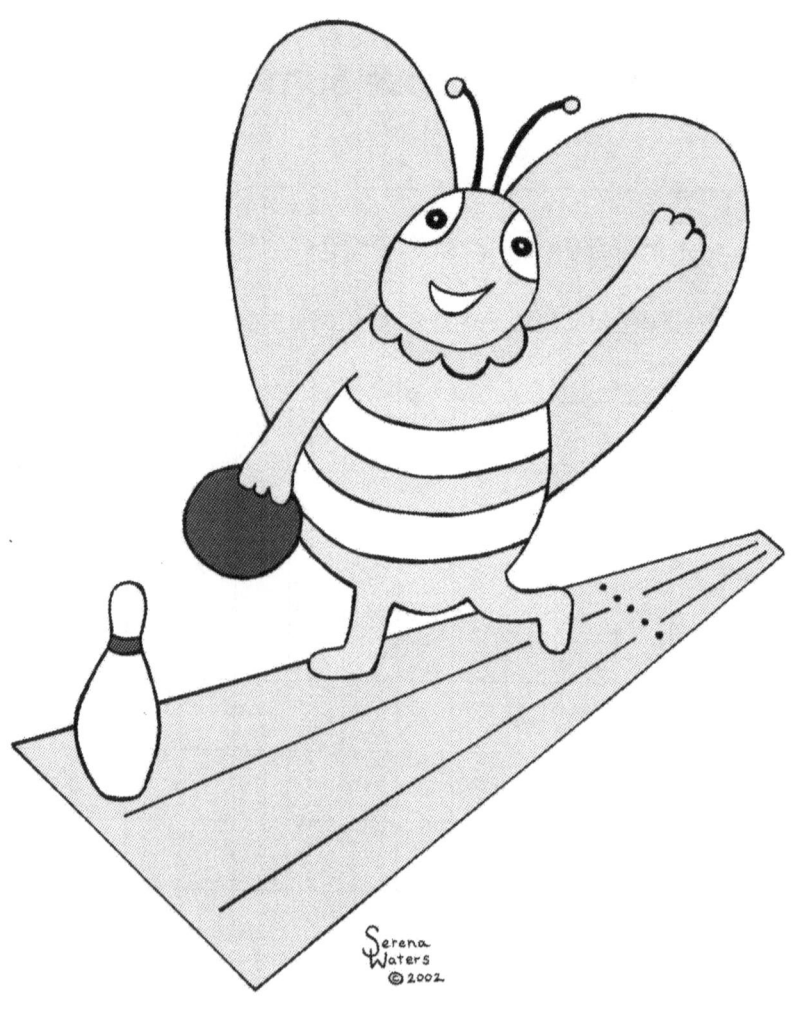

Bee ready for fun! Do what makes you happy!

Time	Monday,_____ Meals and snacks	Carbs or Exchanges	Glucose Reading Pre	Post	Insulin	Meds

Carbohydrates / Exchanges _____ Total _____ Goal

Journal your exercise, thoughts or feelings here.   Ketones _____

_____

_____

_____

Time	**Tuesday,**_____ Meals and snacks	Carbs or Exchanges	Glucose Reading		Insulin	Meds
			Pre	Post		

Carbohydrates / Exchanges _____ **Total** _____ **Goal**

Journal your exercise, thoughts or feelings here.   Ketones _____

_____

_____

_____

Time	Wednesday,_____ Meals and snacks	Carbs or Exchanges	Glucose Reading		Insulin	Meds
			Pre	Post		

Carbohydrates / Exchanges _____ **Total** _____ **Goal**

Journal your exercise, thoughts or feelings here.　　　　Ketones _____

_____
_____
_____

Time	Thursday,_____ Meals and snacks	Carbs or Exchanges	Glucose Reading Pre	Post	Insulin	Meds

Carbohydrates / Exchanges _____ **Total** _____ **Goal**

Journal your exercise, thoughts or feelings here.   Ketones _____

_____

_____

_____

Time	Friday,_____ Meals and snacks	Carbs or Exchanges	Glucose Reading		Insulin	Meds
			Pre	Post		
Carbohydrates / Exchanges _____ **Total** _____ **Goal**						

Journal your exercise, thoughts or feelings here.   Ketones _____

_____

_____

_____

Time	Saturday,_____ Meals and snacks	Carbs or Exchanges	Glucose Reading		Insulin	Meds
			Pre	Post		

Carbohydrates / Exchanges _____ **Total** _____ **Goal**

Journal your exercise, thoughts or feelings here.   Ketones _____

_____

_____

_____

Time	Sunday,_____ Meals and snacks	Carbs or Exchanges	Glucose Reading		Insulin	Meds
			Pre	Post		

Carbohydrates / Exchanges _____ **Total** _____ **Goal**

Journal your exercise, thoughts or feelings here.　　　　Ketones _____

_____

_____

_____

Week of _____

Blood Glucose Summary

Time	Mon		Tues		Wed		Thurs		Fri		Sat		Sun	
	Pre	Post	Pre	Post	Pre	Post	Pre	Post	Pre	Post	Pre	Post	Pre	Post
Average														

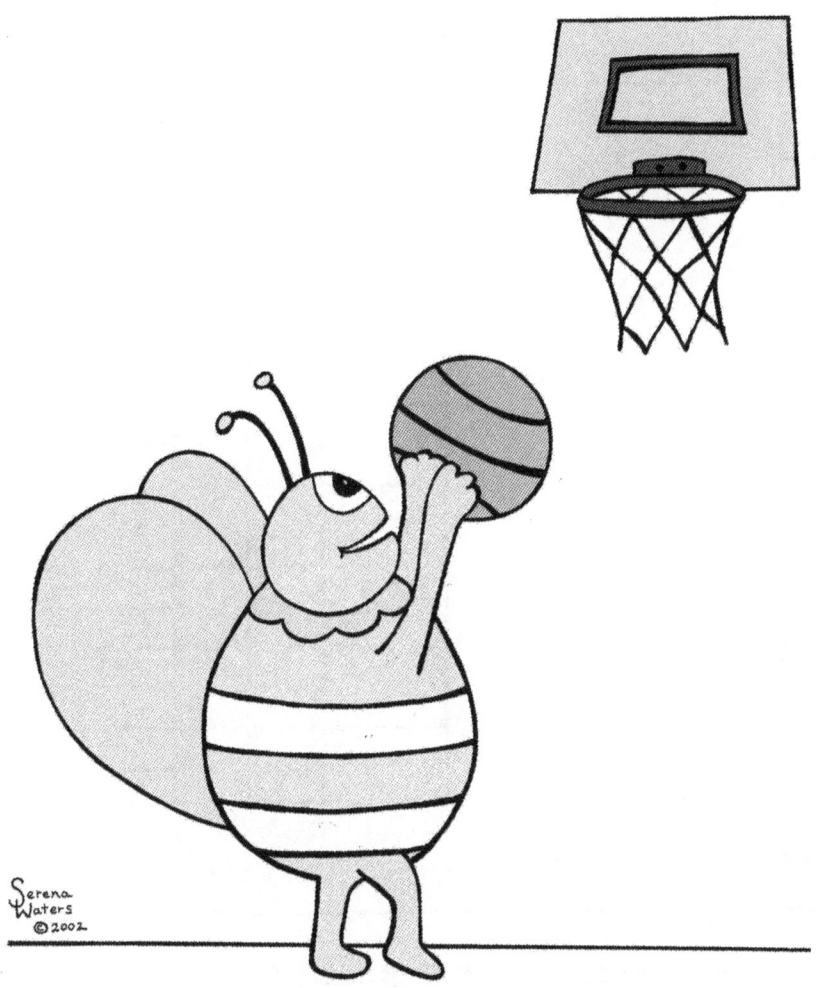

Concentrate! Focus on reaching your goals for health.

Time	Monday,_____ Meals and snacks	Carbs or Exchanges	Glucose Reading		Insulin	Meds
			Pre	Post		

Carbohydrates / Exchanges _____ Total _____ Goal

Journal your exercise, thoughts or feelings here.   Ketones _____

_____

_____

_____

Time	Tuesday,_____ Meals and snacks	Carbs or Exchanges	Glucose Reading		Insulin	Meds
			Pre	Post		
Carbohydrates / Exchanges _____ Total _____ Goal						

Journal your exercise, thoughts or feelings here.   Ketones _____

_____

_____

_____

Time	Wednesday,_____ Meals and snacks	Carbs or Exchanges	Glucose Reading		Insulin	Meds
			Pre	Post		

Carbohydrates / Exchanges _____ **Total** _____ **Goal**

Journal your exercise, thoughts or feelings here.   Ketones _____

_____

_____

_____

Time	Thursday,_____ Meals and snacks	Carbs or Exchanges	Glucose Reading		Insulin	Meds
			Pre	Post		

Carbohydrates / Exchanges _____ **Total** _____ **Goal**

Journal your exercise, thoughts or feelings here.   Ketones _____

_____

_____

_____

Time	Friday,_____ Meals and snacks	Carbs or Exchanges	Glucose Reading Pre	Post	Insulin	Meds

Carbohydrates / Exchanges _____ Total _____ Goal

Journal your exercise, thoughts or feelings here.   Ketones _____

_____

_____

_____

Time	Saturday,_____ Meals and snacks	Carbs or Exchanges	Glucose Reading		Insulin	Meds
			Pre	Post		

Carbohydrates / Exchanges _____ Total _____ Goal

Journal your exercise, thoughts or feelings here.　　　Ketones _____

_____

_____

_____

Time	Sunday,_____ Meals and snacks	Carbs or Exchanges	Glucose Reading		Insulin	Meds
			Pre	Post		

Carbohydrates / Exchanges _____ **Total** _____ **Goal**

Journal your exercise, thoughts or feelings here.   Ketones _____

_____

_____

_____

Week of _____

Blood Glucose Summary

Time	Mon		Tues		Wed		Thurs		Fri		Sat		Sun	
	Pre	Post	Pre	Post	Pre	Post	Pre	Post	Pre	Post	Pre	Post	Pre	Post
Average														

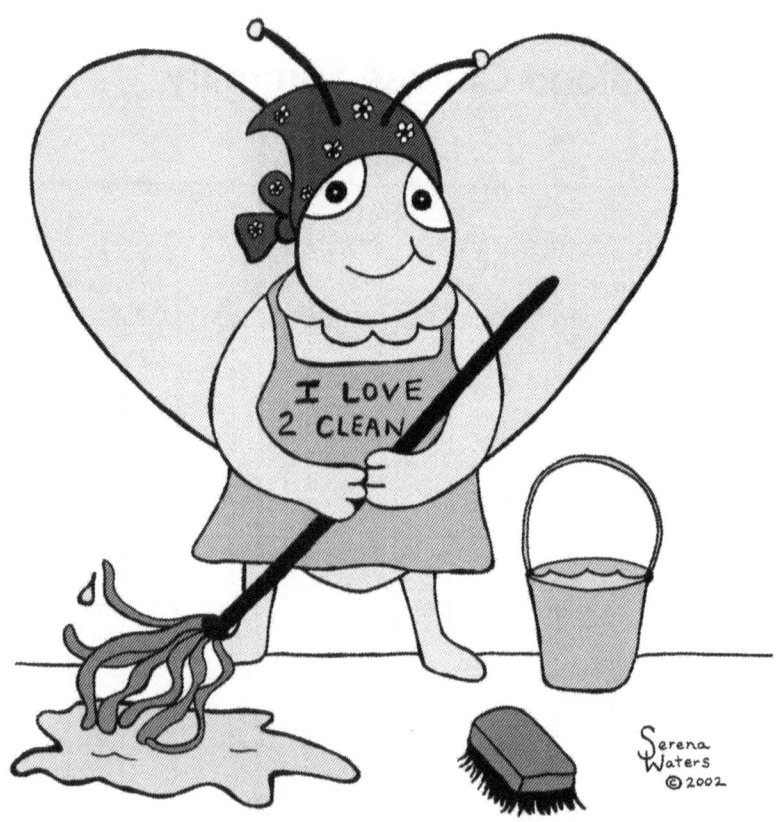

Be active! Your body is designed for moving.

Time	**Monday,**_____ Meals and snacks	Carbs or Exchanges	Glucose Reading		Insulin	Meds
			Pre	Post		
Carbohydrates / Exchanges _____ **Total** _____ **Goal**						

Journal your exercise, thoughts or feelings here.   Ketones _____

_____
_____
_____

Time	Tuesday,_____ Meals and snacks	Carbs or Exchanges	Glucose Reading		Insulin	Meds
			Pre	Post		
Carbohydrates / Exchanges _____ **Total** _____ **Goal**						

Journal your exercise, thoughts or feelings here.   Ketones _____

_____
_____
_____

Time	Wednesday,_____ Meals and snacks	Carbs or Exchanges	Glucose Reading		Insulin	Meds
			Pre	Post		

Carbohydrates / Exchanges _____ Total _____ Goal

Journal your exercise, thoughts or feelings here.   Ketones _____

_____
_____
_____

Time	Thursday,_____ Meals and snacks	Carbs or Exchanges	Glucose Reading		Insulin	Meds
			Pre	Post		

Carbohydrates / Exchanges _____ Total _____ Goal

Journal your exercise, thoughts or feelings here.   Ketones _____

_____
_____
_____

Time	Friday,_____ Meals and snacks	Carbs or Exchanges	Glucose Reading Pre	Post	Insulin	Meds

Carbohydrates / Exchanges _____ Total _____ Goal

Journal your exercise, thoughts or feelings here.   Ketones _____

_____
_____
_____

Time	Saturday,_____ Meals and snacks	Carbs or Exchanges	Glucose Reading		Insulin	Meds
			Pre	Post		

Carbohydrates / Exchanges _____ **Total** _____ **Goal**

Journal your exercise, thoughts or feelings here.   Ketones _____

_____

_____

_____

Time	Sunday,_____ Meals and snacks	Carbs or Exchanges	Glucose Reading Pre | Post		Insulin	Meds
Carbohydrates / Exchanges _____ Total _____ Goal						

Journal your exercise, thoughts or feelings here.   Ketones _____

_____
_____
_____

Week of _____

Blood Glucose Summary

Time	Mon		Tues		Wed		Thurs		Fri		Sat		Sun	
	Pre	Post	Pre	Post	Pre	Post	Pre	Post	Pre	Post	Pre	Post	Pre	Post
Average														

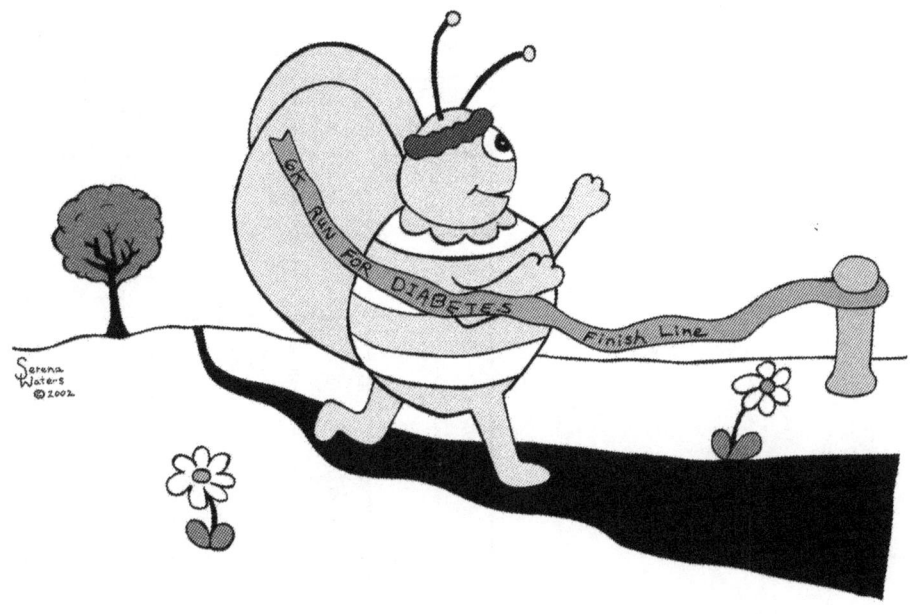

*Bee*lieve in yourself!

Time	Monday,_____ Meals and snacks	Carbs or Exchanges	Glucose Reading		Insulin	Meds
			Pre	Post		

Carbohydrates / Exchanges _____ **Total** _____ **Goal**

Journal your exercise, thoughts or feelings here.   Ketones _____

_____

_____

_____

Time	Tuesday,_____ Meals and snacks	Carbs or Exchanges	Glucose Reading		Insulin	Meds
			Pre	Post		

Carbohydrates / Exchanges _____ **Total** _____ **Goal**

Journal your exercise, thoughts or feelings here.   Ketones _____

_____

_____

_____

Time	Wednesday,_____ Meals and snacks	Carbs or Exchanges	Glucose Reading		Insulin	Meds
			Pre	Post		

Carbohydrates / Exchanges _____ **Total** _____ **Goal**

Journal your exercise, thoughts or feelings here.   Ketones _____

_____

_____

_____

Time	Thursday,_____ Meals and snacks	Carbs or Exchanges	Glucose Reading		Insulin	Meds
			Pre	Post		

Carbohydrates / Exchanges _____ **Total** _____ **Goal**

Journal your exercise, thoughts or feelings here.   Ketones _____

_____

_____

_____

Time	Friday,_____ Meals and snacks	Carbs or Exchanges	Glucose Reading		Insulin	Meds
			Pre	Post		
Carbohydrates / Exchanges _____ **Total** _____ **Goal**						

Journal your exercise, thoughts or feelings here.   Ketones _____

_____

_____

_____

Time	Saturday,_____ Meals and snacks	Carbs or Exchanges	Glucose Reading Pre	Post	Insulin	Meds

Carbohydrates / Exchanges _____ **Total** _____ **Goal**

Journal your exercise, thoughts or feelings here.   Ketones _____

_____

_____

_____

Time	Sunday,_____ Meals and snacks	Carbs or Exchanges	Glucose Reading		Insulin	Meds
			Pre	Post		

Carbohydrates / Exchanges _____ **Total** _____ **Goal**

Journal your exercise, thoughts or feelings here.   Ketones _____

_____

_____

_____

Week of _____

Blood Glucose Summary

Time	Mon		Tues		Wed		Thurs		Fri		Sat		Sun	
	Pre	Post	Pre	Post	Pre	Post	Pre	Post	Pre	Post	Pre	Post	Pre	Post
Average														

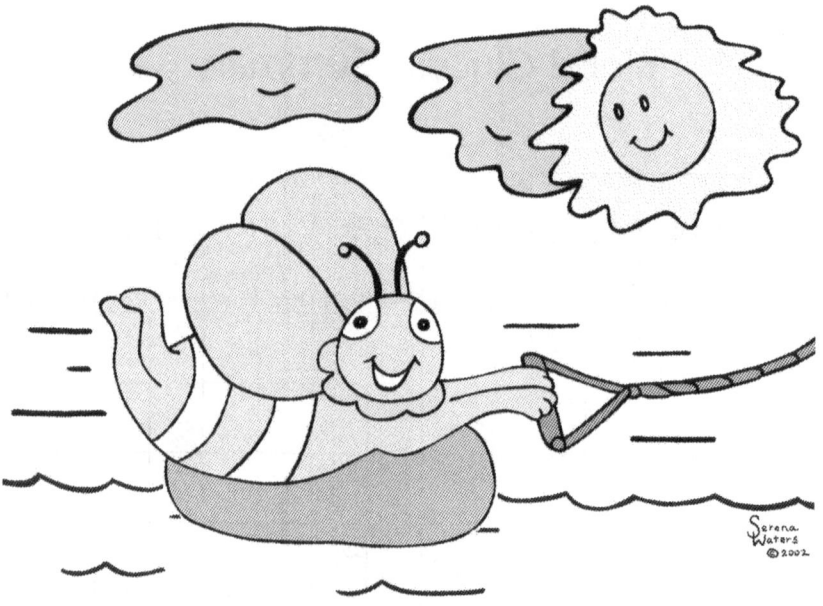

Bee adventurous! Grab onto new opportunities.

Time	Monday,_____ Meals and snacks	Carbs or Exchanges	Glucose Reading		Insulin	Meds
			Pre	Post		

Carbohydrates / Exchanges _____ Total _____ Goal

Journal your exercise, thoughts or feelings here.   Ketones _____

_____

_____

_____

Time	Tuesday,_____ Meals and snacks	Carbs or Exchanges	Glucose Reading		Insulin	Meds
			Pre	Post		

Carbohydrates / Exchanges _____ **Total** _____ **Goal**

Journal your exercise, thoughts or feelings here.   Ketones _____

_____

_____

_____

Time	Wednesday,_____ Meals and snacks	Carbs or Exchanges	Glucose Reading Pre	Post	Insulin	Meds

Carbohydrates / Exchanges _____ **Total** _____ **Goal**

Journal your exercise, thoughts or feelings here.   Ketones _____

_____

_____

_____

Time	Thursday,_____ Meals and snacks	Carbs or Exchanges	Glucose Reading		Insulin	Meds
			Pre	Post		

Carbohydrates / Exchanges _____ Total _____ Goal

Journal your exercise, thoughts or feelings here.   Ketones _____

_____

_____

_____

Time	Friday,_____ Meals and snacks	Carbs or Exchanges	Glucose Reading		Insulin	Meds
			Pre	Post		

Carbohydrates / Exchanges _____ **Total** _____ **Goal**

Journal your exercise, thoughts or feelings here.   Ketones _____

_____

_____

_____

Time	Saturday,_____ Meals and snacks	Carbs or Exchanges	Glucose Reading		Insulin	Meds
			Pre	Post		

Carbohydrates / Exchanges _____ **Total** _____ **Goal**

Journal your exercise, thoughts or feelings here.   Ketones _____

_____

_____

_____

Time	Sunday,_____ Meals and snacks	Carbs or Exchanges	Glucose Reading		Insulin	Meds
			Pre	Post		

Carbohydrates / Exchanges _____ Total _____ Goal

Journal your exercise, thoughts or feelings here.   Ketones _____

_____

_____

_____

Week of _____

Blood Glucose Summary

Time	Mon		Tues		Wed		Thurs		Fri		Sat		Sun	
	Pre	Post	Pre	Post	Pre	Post	Pre	Post	Pre	Post	Pre	Post	Pre	Post
Average														

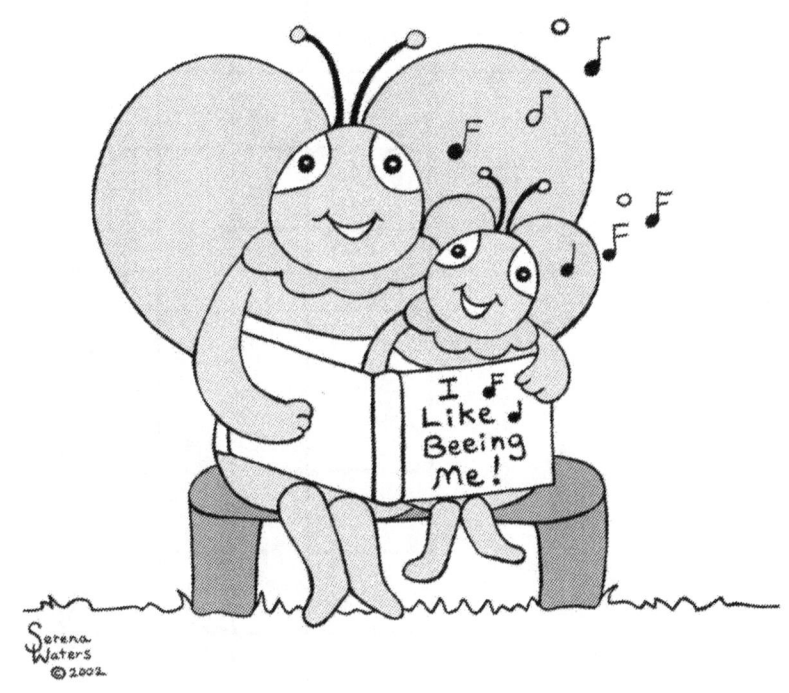

You are a unique note,
a divine part of life's symphony.

Time	Monday,_____ Meals and snacks	Carbs or Exchanges	Glucose Reading		Insulin	Meds
			Pre	Post		

Carbohydrates / Exchanges _____ Total _____ Goal

Journal your exercise, thoughts or feelings here.   Ketones _____

_____
_____
_____

Time	Tuesday,_____ Meals and snacks	Carbs or Exchanges	Glucose Reading		Insulin	Meds
			Pre	Post		
Carbohydrates / Exchanges _____ **Total** _____ **Goal**						

Journal your exercise, thoughts or feelings here.   Ketones _____

_____
_____
_____

Time	Wednesday,_____ Meals and snacks	Carbs or Exchanges	Glucose Reading		Insulin	Meds
			Pre	Post		

Carbohydrates / Exchanges _____ **Total** _____ **Goal**

Journal your exercise, thoughts or feelings here.   Ketones _____

_____
_____
_____

Time	Thursday,_____ Meals and snacks	Carbs or Exchanges	Glucose Reading		Insulin	Meds
			Pre	Post		

Carbohydrates / Exchanges _____ Total _____ Goal

Journal your exercise, thoughts or feelings here.   Ketones _____

_____
_____
_____

Time	Friday,_____ Meals and snacks	Carbs or Exchanges	Glucose Reading		Insulin	Meds
			Pre	Post		

Carbohydrates / Exchanges _____ Total _____ Goal

Journal your exercise, thoughts or feelings here.   Ketones _____

_____

_____

_____

Time	Saturday,_____ Meals and snacks	Carbs or Exchanges	Glucose Reading Pre	Glucose Reading Post	Insulin	Meds

Carbohydrates / Exchanges _____ Total _____ Goal

Journal your exercise, thoughts or feelings here.　　　Ketones _____

_____

_____

_____

Time	Sunday,_____ Meals and snacks	Carbs or Exchanges	Glucose Reading		Insulin	Meds
			Pre	Post		

Carbohydrates / Exchanges _____ **Total** _____ **Goal**

Journal your exercise, thoughts or feelings here.   Ketones _____

_____

_____

_____

Week of _____

Blood Glucose Summary

Time	Mon		Tues		Wed		Thurs		Fri		Sat		Sun	
	Pre	Post	Pre	Post	Pre	Post	Pre	Post	Pre	Post	Pre	Post	Pre	Post
Average														

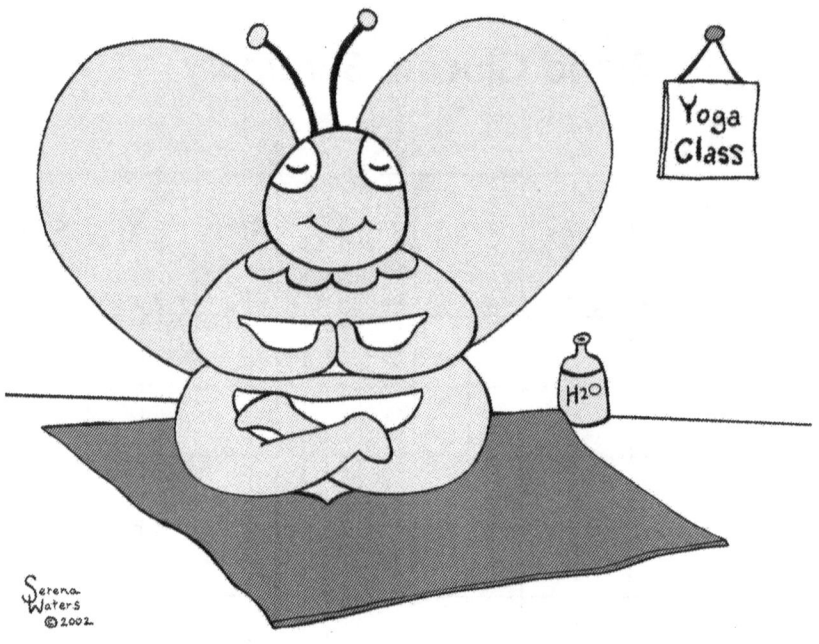

Bee still. Peace comes from knowing your center.

Time	Monday,_____ Meals and snacks	Carbs or Exchanges	Glucose Reading		Insulin	Meds
			Pre	Post		

Carbohydrates / Exchanges _____ **Total** _____ **Goal**

Journal your exercise, thoughts or feelings here.   Ketones _____

_____

_____

_____

Time	Tuesday,_____ Meals and snacks	Carbs or Exchanges	Glucose Reading		Insulin	Meds
			Pre	Post		
Carbohydrates / Exchanges _____ Total _____ Goal						

Journal your exercise, thoughts or feelings here.   Ketones _____

_____

_____

_____

Time	Wednesday,_____ Meals and snacks	Carbs or Exchanges	Glucose Reading		Insulin	Meds
			Pre	Post		
Carbohydrates / Exchanges _____ Total _____ Goal						

Journal your exercise, thoughts or feelings here.   Ketones _____

_____
_____
_____

Time	Thursday,_____ Meals and snacks	Carbs or Exchanges	Glucose Reading Pre	Post	Insulin	Meds

Carbohydrates / Exchanges _____ **Total** _____ **Goal**

Journal your exercise, thoughts or feelings here.   Ketones _____

_____

_____

_____

Time	Friday,_____ Meals and snacks	Carbs or Exchanges	Glucose Reading Pre	Post	Insulin	Meds

Carbohydrates / Exchanges _____ **Total** _____ **Goal**

Journal your exercise, thoughts or feelings here.   Ketones _____

_____

_____

_____

Time	Saturday,_____ Meals and snacks	Carbs or Exchanges	Glucose Reading		Insulin	Meds
			Pre	Post		

Carbohydrates / Exchanges _____ Total _____ Goal

Journal your exercise, thoughts or feelings here.   Ketones _____

_____

_____

_____

Time	Sunday,_____ Meals and snacks	Carbs or Exchanges	Glucose Reading		Insulin	Meds
			Pre	Post		

Carbohydrates / Exchanges _____ Total _____ Goal

Journal your exercise, thoughts or feelings here.   Ketones _____

_____
_____
_____

Week of _____

Blood Glucose Summary

Time	Mon		Tues		Wed		Thurs		Fri		Sat		Sun	
	Pre	Post	Pre	Post	Pre	Post	Pre	Post	Pre	Post	Pre	Post	Pre	Post
Average														

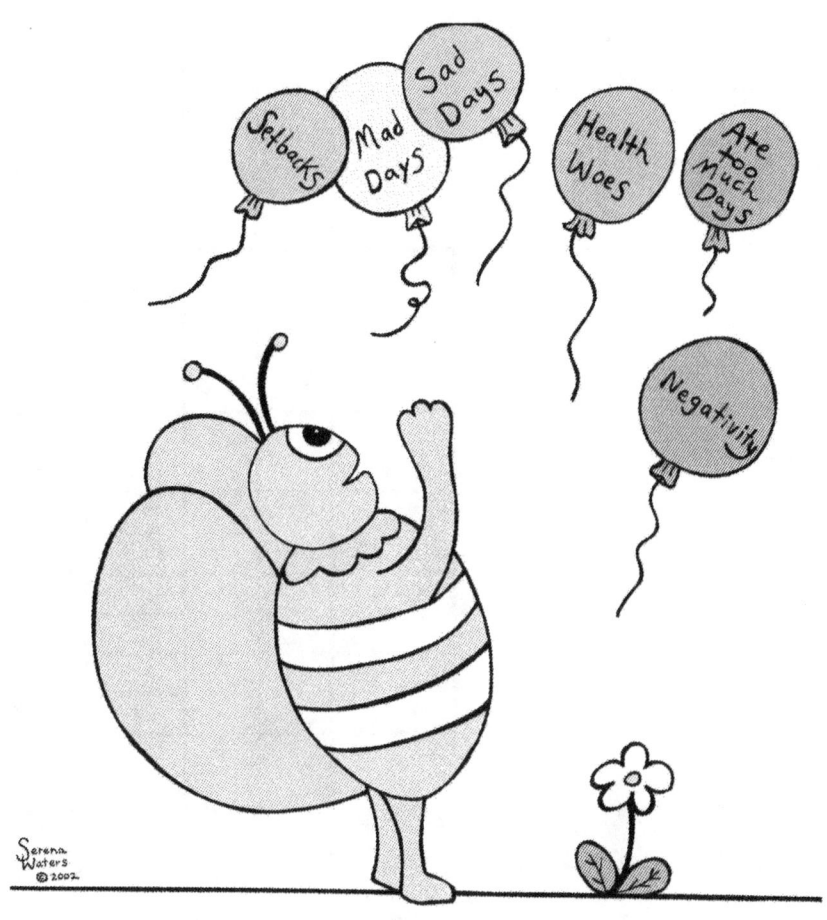

Bee free! Release the past. Embrace the future.

Time	Monday,_____ Meals and snacks	Carbs or Exchanges	Glucose Reading		Insulin	Meds
			Pre	Post		
Carbohydrates / Exchanges _____ **Total** _____ **Goal**						

Journal your exercise, thoughts or feelings here.   Ketones _____

_____

_____

_____

Time	Tuesday,_____ Meals and snacks	Carbs or Exchanges	Glucose Reading		Insulin	Meds
			Pre	Post		

Carbohydrates / Exchanges _____ **Total** _____ **Goal**

Journal your exercise, thoughts or feelings here.   Ketones _____

_____
_____
_____

Time	Wednesday,_____ Meals and snacks	Carbs or Exchanges	Glucose Reading		Insulin	Meds
			Pre	Post		
Carbohydrates / Exchanges _____ **Total** _____ **Goal**						

Journal your exercise, thoughts or feelings here.   Ketones _____

_____

_____

_____

Time	Thursday,_____ Meals and snacks	Carbs or Exchanges	Glucose Reading Pre	Post	Insulin	Meds
Carbohydrates / Exchanges _____ Total _____ Goal						

Journal your exercise, thoughts or feelings here.   Ketones _____

_____

_____

_____

Time	Friday,_____ Meals and snacks	Carbs or Exchanges	Glucose Reading		Insulin	Meds
			Pre	Post		
Carbohydrates / Exchanges _____ **Total** _____ **Goal**						

Journal your exercise, thoughts or feelings here.   Ketones _____

_____

_____

_____

Time	Saturday,_____ Meals and snacks	Carbs or Exchanges	Glucose Reading		Insulin	Meds
			Pre	Post		
Carbohydrates / Exchanges _____ Total _____ Goal						

Journal your exercise, thoughts or feelings here.   Ketones _____

_____
_____
_____

Time	Sunday,_____ Meals and snacks	Carbs or Exchanges	Glucose Reading		Insulin	Meds
			Pre	Post		

Carbohydrates / Exchanges _____ **Total** _____ **Goal**

Journal your exercise, thoughts or feelings here.   Ketones _____

_____

_____

_____

Week of _____

Blood Glucose Summary

Time	Mon		Tues		Wed		Thurs		Fri		Sat		Sun	
	Pre	Post	Pre	Post	Pre	Post	Pre	Post	Pre	Post	Pre	Post	Pre	Post
Average														

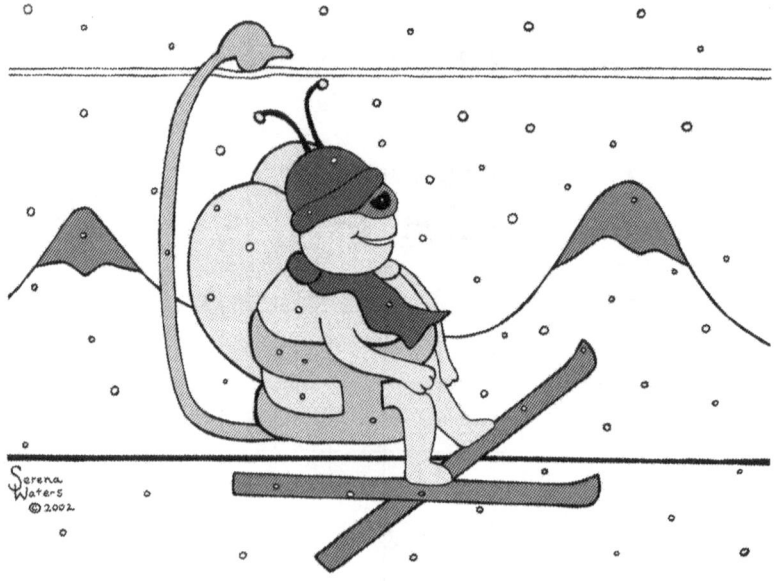

Bee brave! The view is beautiful from the top.

Time	Monday,_____ Meals and snacks	Carbs or Exchanges	Glucose Reading		Insulin	Meds
			Pre	Post		

Carbohydrates / Exchanges _____ Total _____ Goal

Journal your exercise, thoughts or feelings here.   Ketones _____

_____

_____

_____

Time	Tuesday,_____ Meals and snacks	Carbs or Exchanges	Glucose Reading		Insulin	Meds
			Pre	Post		

Carbohydrates / Exchanges _____ **Total** _____ **Goal**

Journal your exercise, thoughts or feelings here.   Ketones _____

_____
_____
_____

Time	Wednesday,_____ Meals and snacks	Carbs or Exchanges	Glucose Reading		Insulin	Meds
			Pre	Post		

Carbohydrates / Exchanges _____ **Total** _____ **Goal**

Journal your exercise, thoughts or feelings here.   Ketones _____

_____
_____
_____

Time	Thursday,_____ Meals and snacks	Carbs or Exchanges	Glucose Reading		Insulin	Meds
			Pre	Post		

Carbohydrates / Exchanges _____ Total _____ Goal

Journal your exercise, thoughts or feelings here.   Ketones _____

_____

_____

_____

Time	Friday,_____ Meals and snacks	Carbs or Exchanges	Glucose Reading		Insulin	Meds
			Pre	Post		

Carbohydrates / Exchanges _____ Total _____ Goal

Journal your exercise, thoughts or feelings here.   Ketones _____

_____

_____

_____

Time	Saturday,_____ Meals and snacks	Carbs or Exchanges	Glucose Reading Pre	Post	Insulin	Meds

Carbohydrates / Exchanges _____ Total _____ Goal

Journal your exercise, thoughts or feelings here.   Ketones _____

_____

_____

_____

Time	Sunday,_____ Meals and snacks	Carbs or Exchanges	Glucose Reading		Insulin	Meds
			Pre	Post		

Carbohydrates / Exchanges _____ **Total** _____ **Goal**

Journal your exercise, thoughts or feelings here.   Ketones _____

_____
_____
_____

Week of _____

Blood Glucose Summary

Time	Mon		Tues		Wed		Thurs		Fri		Sat		Sun	
	Pre	Post	Pre	Post	Pre	Post	Pre	Post	Pre	Post	Pre	Post	Pre	Post
Average														

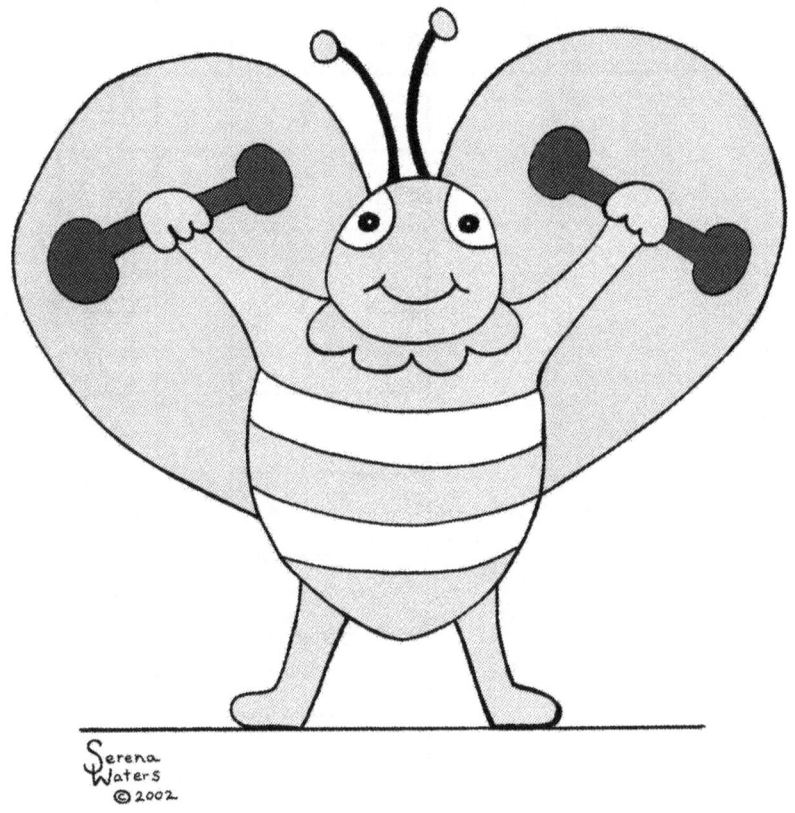

Serena
Waters
© 2002

Bee strong! The seeds of strength grow inside you.

Time	Monday,_____ Meals and snacks	Carbs or Exchanges	Glucose Reading		Insulin	Meds
			Pre	Post		

Carbohydrates / Exchanges _____ **Total** _____ **Goal**

Journal your exercise, thoughts or feelings here.   Ketones _____

_____

_____

_____

Time	Tuesday,_____ Meals and snacks	Carbs or Exchanges	Glucose Reading		Insulin	Meds
			Pre	Post		

Carbohydrates / Exchanges _____ **Total** _____ **Goal**

Journal your exercise, thoughts or feelings here.   Ketones _____

_____
_____
_____

125

Time	Wednesday,_____ Meals and snacks	Carbs or Exchanges	Glucose Reading Pre	Glucose Reading Post	Insulin	Meds

Carbohydrates / Exchanges _____ Total _____ Goal

Journal your exercise, thoughts or feelings here.   Ketones _____

_____
_____
_____

Time	Thursday,_____ Meals and snacks	Carbs or Exchanges	Glucose Reading		Insulin	Meds
			Pre	Post		
Carbohydrates / Exchanges _____ Total _____ Goal						

Journal your exercise, thoughts or feelings here.   Ketones _____

_____

_____

_____

Time	Friday,_____ Meals and snacks	Carbs or Exchanges	Glucose Reading Pre	Post	Insulin	Meds

Carbohydrates / Exchanges _____ **Total** _____ **Goal**

Journal your exercise, thoughts or feelings here.   Ketones _____

_____

_____

_____

Time	Saturday,_____ Meals and snacks	Carbs or Exchanges	Glucose Reading		Insulin	Meds
			Pre	Post		
Carbohydrates / Exchanges _____ **Total**				_____ **Goal**		

Journal your exercise, thoughts or feelings here.   Ketones _____

_____

_____

_____

Time	Sunday,_____ Meals and snacks	Carbs or Exchanges	Glucose Reading		Insulin	Meds
			Pre	Post		

Carbohydrates / Exchanges _____ **Total** _____ **Goal**

Journal your exercise, thoughts or feelings here.   Ketones _____

_____

_____

_____

Week of _____

Blood Glucose Summary

Time	Mon		Tues		Wed		Thurs		Fri		Sat		Sun	
	Pre	Post	Pre	Post	Pre	Post	Pre	Post	Pre	Post	Pre	Post	Pre	Post
Average														

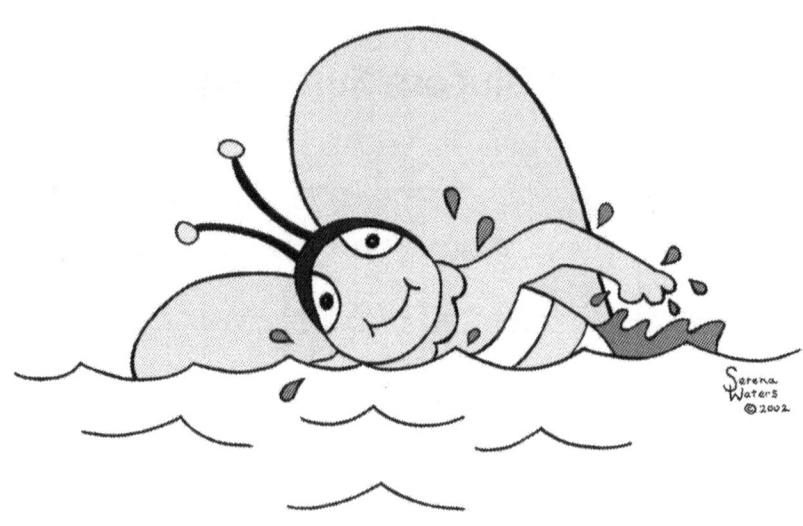

Bee consistent! Success is doing it. Do it again!

Time	Monday,_____ Meals and snacks	Carbs or Exchanges	Glucose Reading		Insulin	Meds
			Pre	Post		
Carbohydrates / Exchanges _____ **Total** _____ **Goal**						

Journal your exercise, thoughts or feelings here.   Ketones _____

_____
_____
_____

Time	Tuesday,_____ Meals and snacks	Carbs or Exchanges	Glucose Reading		Insulin	Meds
			Pre	Post		

Carbohydrates / Exchanges _____ Total _____ Goal

Journal your exercise, thoughts or feelings here.   Ketones _____

_____

_____

_____

Time	Wednesday,_____ Meals and snacks	Carbs or Exchanges	Glucose Reading		Insulin	Meds
			Pre	Post		
Carbohydrates / Exchanges _____ Total _____ Goal						

Journal your exercise, thoughts or feelings here.   Ketones _____

_____

_____

_____

Time	Thursday,_____ Meals and snacks	Carbs or Exchanges	Glucose Reading		Insulin	Meds
			Pre	Post		

Carbohydrates / Exchanges _____ **Total** _____ **Goal**

Journal your exercise, thoughts or feelings here.   Ketones _____

_____

_____

_____

Time	Friday,_____ Meals and snacks	Carbs or Exchanges	Glucose Reading		Insulin	Meds
			Pre	Post		
Carbohydrates / Exchanges _____ **Total** _____ **Goal**						

Journal your exercise, thoughts or feelings here.   Ketones _____

_____

_____

_____

Time	Saturday,_____ Meals and snacks	Carbs or Exchanges	Glucose Reading Pre	Post	Insulin	Meds

Carbohydrates / Exchanges _____ Total _____ Goal

Journal your exercise, thoughts or feelings here.   Ketones _____

_____

_____

_____

Time	Sunday,_____ Meals and snacks	Carbs or Exchanges	Glucose Reading		Insulin	Meds
			Pre	Post		

Carbohydrates / Exchanges _____ **Total** _____ **Goal**

Journal your exercise, thoughts or feelings here.   Ketones _____

_____

_____

_____

Week of _____

Blood Glucose Summary

Time	Mon		Tues		Wed		Thurs		Fri		Sat		Sun	
	Pre	Post	Pre	Post	Pre	Post	Pre	Post	Pre	Post	Pre	Post	Pre	Post
Average														

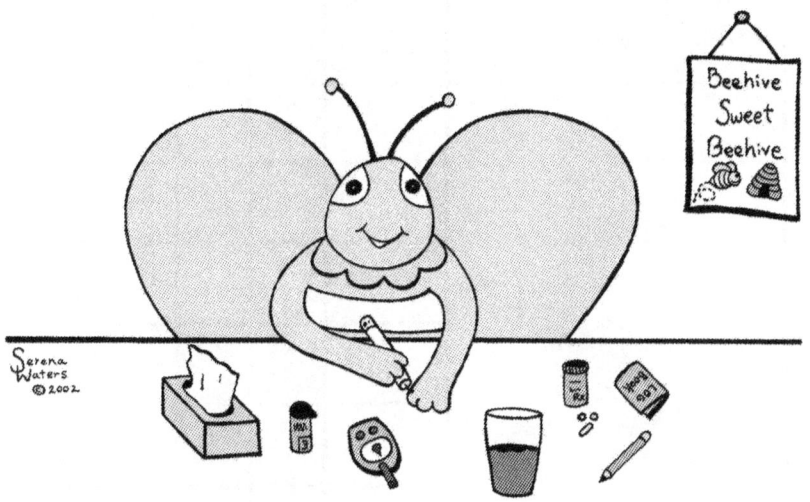

Test regularly! The benefits are in the knowing.

Time	Monday,_____ Meals and snacks	Carbs or Exchanges	Glucose Reading		Insulin	Meds
			Pre	Post		
Carbohydrates / Exchanges _____ **Total** _____ **Goal**						

Journal your exercise, thoughts or feelings here.   Ketones _____

_____

_____

_____

Time	Tuesday,_____ Meals and snacks	Carbs or Exchanges	Glucose Reading		Insulin	Meds
			Pre	Post		

Carbohydrates / Exchanges _____ **Total** _____ **Goal**

Journal your exercise, thoughts or feelings here.   Ketones _____

_____
_____
_____

Time	Wednesday,_____ Meals and snacks	Carbs or Exchanges	Glucose Reading		Insulin	Meds
			Pre	Post		
Carbohydrates / Exchanges _____ **Total** _____ **Goal**						

Journal your exercise, thoughts or feelings here.   Ketones _____

_____

_____

_____

Time	Thursday,_____ Meals and snacks	Carbs or Exchanges	Glucose Reading Pre	Glucose Reading Post	Insulin	Meds

Carbohydrates / Exchanges _____ Total _____ Goal

Journal your exercise, thoughts or feelings here.   Ketones _____

_____

_____

_____

145

Time	Friday,_____ Meals and snacks	Carbs or Exchanges	Glucose Reading		Insulin	Meds
			Pre	Post		

Carbohydrates / Exchanges _____ Total _____ Goal

Journal your exercise, thoughts or feelings here.   Ketones _____

_____

_____

_____

Time	Saturday,_____ Meals and snacks	Carbs or Exchanges	Glucose Reading		Insulin	Meds
			Pre	Post		
Carbohydrates / Exchanges _____ **Total** _____ **Goal**						

Journal your exercise, thoughts or feelings here.   Ketones _____

_____

_____

_____

Time	Sunday,_____ Meals and snacks	Carbs or Exchanges	Glucose Reading		Insulin	Meds
			Pre	Post		

Carbohydrates / Exchanges _____ Total _____ Goal

Journal your exercise, thoughts or feelings here.   Ketones _____

_____

_____

_____

Week of _____

Blood Glucose Summary

Time	Mon		Tues		Wed		Thurs		Fri		Sat		Sun	
	Pre	Post	Pre	Post	Pre	Post	Pre	Post	Pre	Post	Pre	Post	Pre	Post
Average														

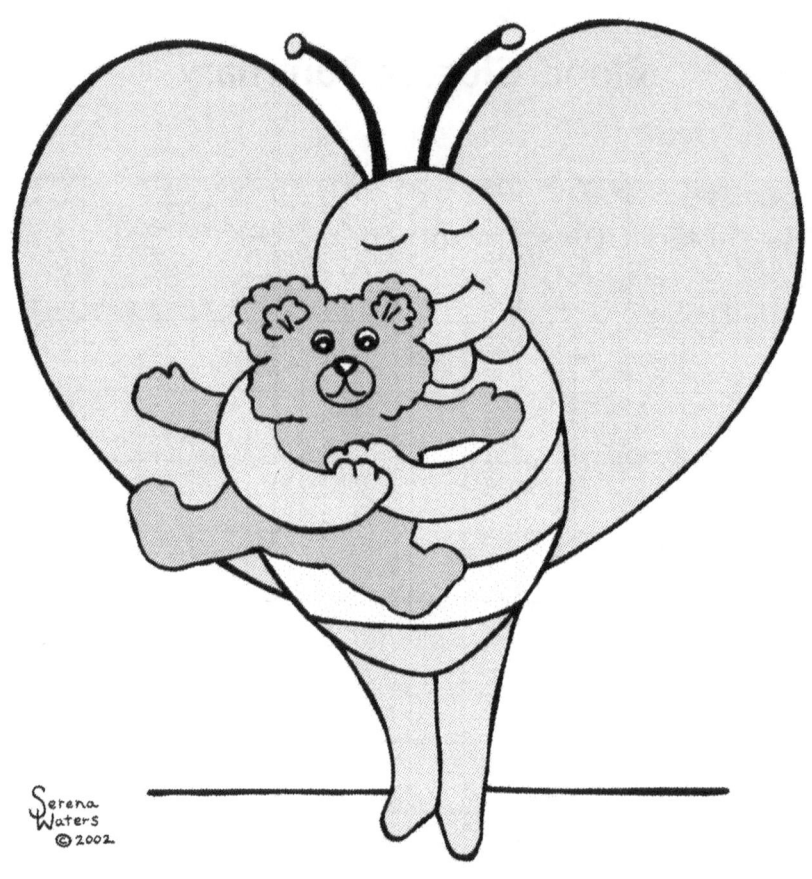

Bee your own Buddy! Hug yourself and embrace life!

Time	Monday,_____ Meals and snacks	Carbs or Exchanges	Glucose Reading		Insulin	Meds
			Pre	Post		

Carbohydrates / Exchanges _____ **Total** _____ **Goal**

Journal your exercise, thoughts or feelings here.   Ketones _____

_____
_____
_____

Time	Tuesday,_____ Meals and snacks	Carbs or Exchanges	Glucose Reading Pre	Post	Insulin	Meds

Carbohydrates / Exchanges _____ **Total** _____ **Goal**

Journal your exercise, thoughts or feelings here.   Ketones _____

_____

_____

_____

Time	Wednesday,_____ Meals and snacks	Carbs or Exchanges	Glucose Reading		Insulin	Meds
			Pre	Post		

Carbohydrates / Exchanges _____ Total _____ Goal

Journal your exercise, thoughts or feelings here.   Ketones _____

_____
_____
_____

Time	Thursday,_____ Meals and snacks	Carbs or Exchanges	Glucose Reading Pre	Post	Insulin	Meds

Carbohydrates / Exchanges _____ **Total** _____ **Goal**

Journal your exercise, thoughts or feelings here.   Ketones _____

_____

_____

_____

Time	Friday,_____ Meals and snacks	Carbs or Exchanges	Glucose Reading		Insulin	Meds
			Pre	Post		

Carbohydrates / Exchanges _____ **Total** _____ **Goal**

Journal your exercise, thoughts or feelings here.　　　　Ketones _____

_____
_____
_____

Time	Saturday,_____ Meals and snacks	Carbs or Exchanges	Glucose Reading		Insulin	Meds
			Pre	Post		

Carbohydrates / Exchanges _____ **Total** _____ **Goal**

Journal your exercise, thoughts or feelings here.   Ketones _____

_____

_____

_____

Time	Sunday,_____ Meals and snacks	Carbs or Exchanges	Glucose Reading		Insulin	Meds
			Pre	Post		

Carbohydrates / Exchanges _____ **Total** _____ **Goal**

Journal your exercise, thoughts or feelings here.   Ketones _____

_____
_____
_____

Week of _____

Blood Glucose Summary

Time	Mon		Tues		Wed		Thurs		Fri		Sat		Sun	
	Pre	Post	Pre	Post	Pre	Post	Pre	Post	Pre	Post	Pre	Post	Pre	Post
Average														

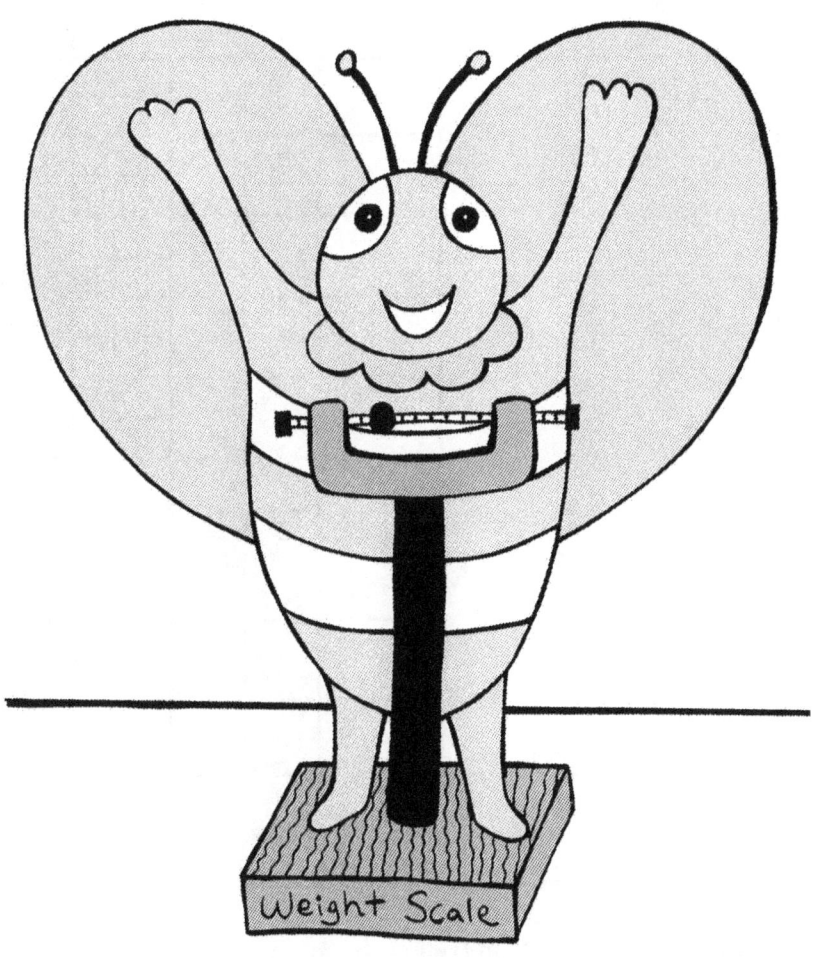

Celebrate the little goals. You can do it!

Time	Monday,_____ Meals and snacks	Carbs or Exchanges	Glucose Reading Pre	Glucose Reading Post	Insulin	Meds

Carbohydrates / Exchanges _____ Total _____ Goal

Journal your exercise, thoughts or feelings here.   Ketones _____

_____

_____

_____

Time	Tuesday,_____ Meals and snacks	Carbs or Exchanges	Glucose Reading		Insulin	Meds
			Pre	Post		
Carbohydrates / Exchanges _____ **Total** _____ **Goal**						

Journal your exercise, thoughts or feelings here.   Ketones _____

_____
_____
_____

Time	Wednesday,_____ Meals and snacks	Carbs or Exchanges	Glucose Reading		Insulin	Meds
			Pre	Post		

Carbohydrates / Exchanges _____ Total _____ Goal

Journal your exercise, thoughts or feelings here.   Ketones _____

_____
_____
_____

Time	Thursday,_____ Meals and snacks	Carbs or Exchanges	Glucose Reading		Insulin	Meds
			Pre	Post		
Carbohydrates / Exchanges _____ Total _____ Goal						

Journal your exercise, thoughts or feelings here.   Ketones _____

_____

_____

_____

Time	Friday,_____ Meals and snacks	Carbs or Exchanges	Glucose Reading		Insulin	Meds
			Pre	Post		

Carbohydrates / Exchanges _____ Total _____ Goal

Journal your exercise, thoughts or feelings here.   Ketones _____

_____

_____

_____

Time	Saturday,_____ Meals and snacks	Carbs or Exchanges	Glucose Reading		Insulin	Meds
			Pre	Post		

Carbohydrates / Exchanges _____ **Total** _____ **Goal**

Journal your exercise, thoughts or feelings here.   Ketones _____

_____

_____

_____

Time	Sunday,_____ Meals and snacks	Carbs or Exchanges	Glucose Reading		Insulin	Meds
			Pre	Post		

Carbohydrates / Exchanges _____ Total _____ Goal

Journal your exercise, thoughts or feelings here.   Ketones _____

_____

_____

_____

Week of _____

Blood Glucose Summary

Time	Mon		Tues		Wed		Thurs		Fri		Sat		Sun	
	Pre	Post	Pre	Post	Pre	Post	Pre	Post	Pre	Post	Pre	Post	Pre	Post
Average														

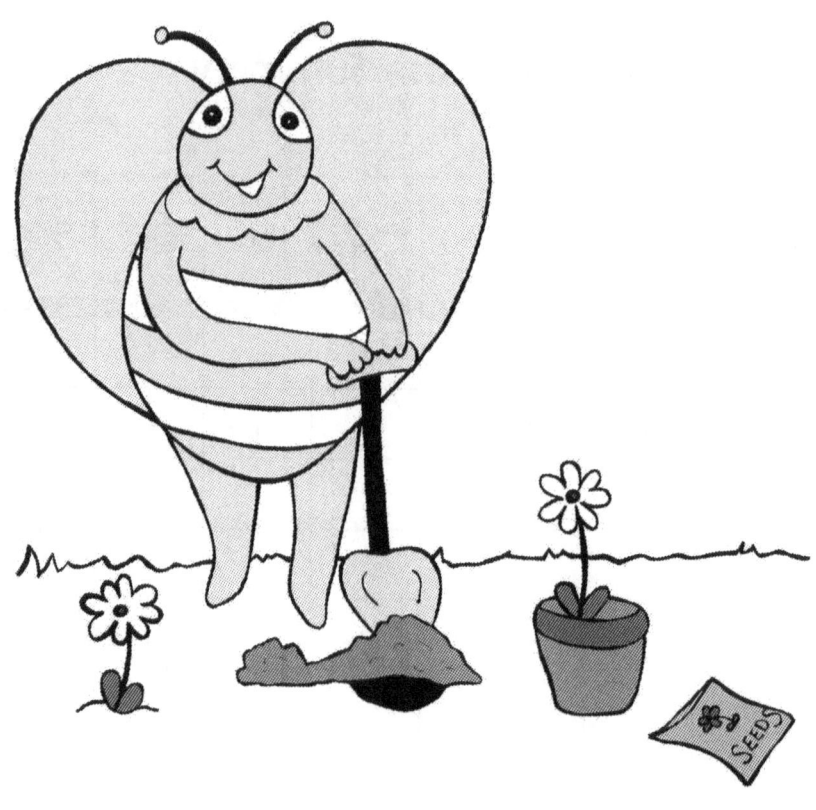

Bee a gardener!
Plant your dreams and goals for health.

Time	Monday,_____ Meals and snacks	Carbs or Exchanges	Glucose Reading		Insulin	Meds
			Pre	Post		

Carbohydrates / Exchanges _____ Total _____ Goal

Journal your exercise, thoughts or feelings here.   Ketones _____

_____

_____

_____

Time	Tuesday,_____ Meals and snacks	Carbs or Exchanges	Glucose Reading		Insulin	Meds
			Pre	Post		

Carbohydrates / Exchanges _____ Total _____ Goal

Journal your exercise, thoughts or feelings here.   Ketones _____

_____

_____

_____

Time	Wednesday,_____ Meals and snacks	Carbs or Exchanges	Glucose Reading		Insulin	Meds
			Pre	Post		
Carbohydrates / Exchanges _____ **Total** _____ **Goal**						

Journal your exercise, thoughts or feelings here.   Ketones _____

_____

_____

_____

Time	Thursday,_____ Meals and snacks	Carbs or Exchanges	Glucose Reading		Insulin	Meds
			Pre	Post		

Carbohydrates / Exchanges _____ **Total** _____ **Goal**

Journal your exercise, thoughts or feelings here.   Ketones _____

_____

_____

_____

Time	Friday,_____ Meals and snacks	Carbs or Exchanges	Glucose Reading		Insulin	Meds
			Pre	Post		
Carbohydrates / Exchanges _____ **Total** _____ **Goal**						

Journal your exercise, thoughts or feelings here.   Ketones _____

_____

_____

_____

Time	Saturday,_____ Meals and snacks	Carbs or Exchanges	Glucose Reading Pre	Glucose Reading Post	Insulin	Meds

Carbohydrates / Exchanges _____ **Total** _____ **Goal**

Journal your exercise, thoughts or feelings here.   Ketones _____

_____

_____

_____

Time	Sunday,_____ Meals and snacks	Carbs or Exchanges	Glucose Reading		Insulin	Meds
			Pre	Post		

Carbohydrates / Exchanges _____ **Total** _____ **Goal**

Journal your exercise, thoughts or feelings here.   Ketones _____

_____
_____
_____

Week of _____

Blood Glucose Summary

Time	Mon		Tues		Wed		Thurs		Fri		Sat		Sun	
	Pre	Post	Pre	Post	Pre	Post	Pre	Post	Pre	Post	Pre	Post	Pre	Post
Average														

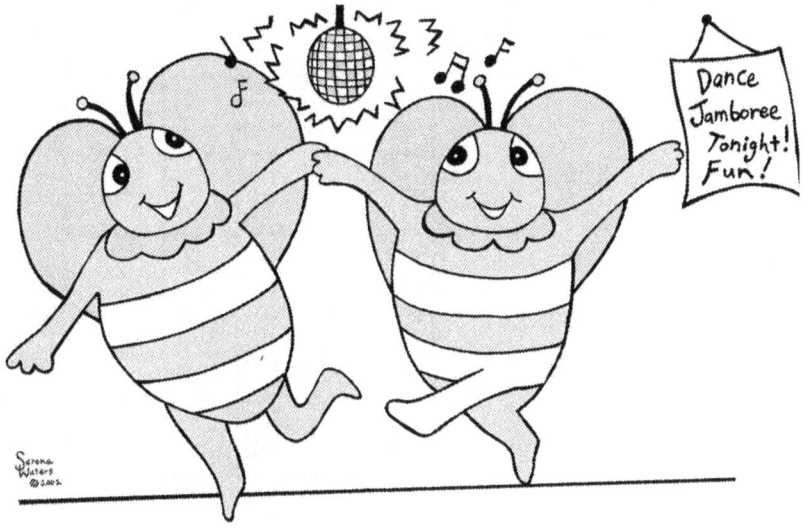

Dance! Let music bee the rhythm that lifts your feet.

Time	Monday,_____ Meals and snacks	Carbs or Exchanges	Glucose Reading		Insulin	Meds
			Pre	Post		
Carbohydrates / Exchanges _____ Total _____ Goal						

Journal your exercise, thoughts or feelings here.   Ketones _____

_____

_____

_____

Time	Tuesday,_____ Meals and snacks	Carbs or Exchanges	Glucose Reading		Insulin	Meds
			Pre	Post		
Carbohydrates / Exchanges _____ **Total** _____ **Goal**						

Journal your exercise, thoughts or feelings here.   Ketones _____

_____
_____
_____

Time	Wednesday,_____ Meals and snacks	Carbs or Exchanges	Glucose Reading		Insulin	Meds
			Pre	Post		

Carbohydrates / Exchanges _____ **Total** _____ **Goal**

Journal your exercise, thoughts or feelings here.   Ketones _____

_____
_____
_____

Time	Thursday,_____ Meals and snacks	Carbs or Exchanges	Glucose Reading		Insulin	Meds
			Pre	Post		
Carbohydrates / Exchanges _____ Total _____ Goal						

Journal your exercise, thoughts or feelings here.   Ketones _____

_____

_____

_____

Time	Friday,_____ Meals and snacks	Carbs or Exchanges	Glucose Reading		Insulin	Meds
			Pre	Post		

Carbohydrates / Exchanges _____ Total _____ Goal

Journal your exercise, thoughts or feelings here.   Ketones _____

_____

_____

_____

Time	Saturday,_____ Meals and snacks	Carbs or Exchanges	Glucose Reading		Insulin	Meds
			Pre	Post		

Carbohydrates / Exchanges _____ **Total** _____ **Goal**

Journal your exercise, thoughts or feelings here.   Ketones _____

_____

_____

_____

Time	Sunday,_____ Meals and snacks	Carbs or Exchanges	Glucose Reading		Insulin	Meds
			Pre	Post		

Carbohydrates / Exchanges _____ **Total** _____ **Goal**

Journal your exercise, thoughts or feelings here.   Ketones _____

_____

_____

_____

Week of _____

Blood Glucose Summary

Time	Mon		Tues		Wed		Thurs		Fri		Sat		Sun	
	Pre	Post	Pre	Post	Pre	Post	Pre	Post	Pre	Post	Pre	Post	Pre	Post
Average														

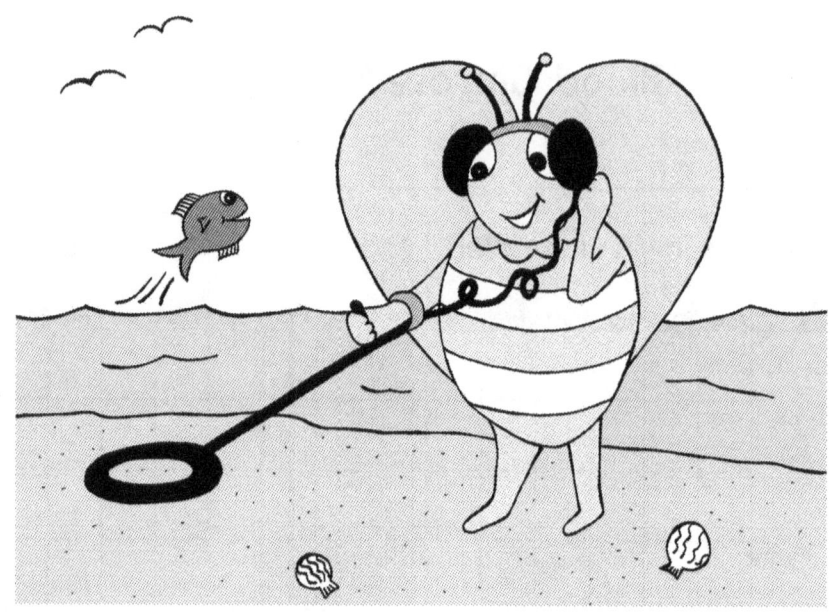

Bee a discoverer! You never know what you may find.

Time	Monday,_____ Meals and snacks	Carbs or Exchanges	Glucose Reading		Insulin	Meds
			Pre	Post		
Carbohydrates / Exchanges _____ **Total** _____ **Goal**						

Journal your exercise, thoughts or feelings here.   Ketones _____

_____
_____
_____

Time	Tuesday,_____ Meals and snacks	Carbs or Exchanges	Glucose Reading		Insulin	Meds
			Pre	Post		

Carbohydrates / Exchanges _____ **Total** _____ **Goal**

Journal your exercise, thoughts or feelings here.　　　　Ketones _____

_____
_____
_____

Time	Wednesday,_____ Meals and snacks	Carbs or Exchanges	Glucose Reading		Insulin	Meds
			Pre	Post		

Carbohydrates / Exchanges _____ Total _____ Goal

Journal your exercise, thoughts or feelings here.   Ketones _____

_____
_____
_____

Time	Thursday,_____ Meals and snacks	Carbs or Exchanges	Glucose Reading		Insulin	Meds
			Pre	Post		

Carbohydrates / Exchanges _____ **Total** _____ **Goal**

Journal your exercise, thoughts or feelings here.   Ketones _____

_____

_____

_____

Time	Friday,_____ Meals and snacks	Carbs or Exchanges	Glucose Reading		Insulin	Meds
			Pre	Post		
Carbohydrates / Exchanges _____ **Total** _____ **Goal**						

Journal your exercise, thoughts or feelings here.   Ketones _____

_____
_____
_____

Time	Saturday,_____ Meals and snacks	Carbs or Exchanges	Glucose Reading		Insulin	Meds
			Pre	Post		

Carbohydrates / Exchanges _____ **Total** _____ **Goal**

Journal your exercise, thoughts or feelings here.   Ketones _____

_____

_____

_____

Time	**Sunday,**_____ Meals and snacks	Carbs or Exchanges	Glucose Reading		Insulin	Meds
			Pre	Post		

Carbohydrates / Exchanges _____ **Total** _____ **Goal**

Journal your exercise, thoughts or feelings here.   Ketones _____

_____
_____
_____

Week of _____

Blood Glucose Summary

Time	Mon		Tues		Wed		Thurs		Fri		Sat		Sun	
	Pre	Post	Pre	Post	Pre	Post	Pre	Post	Pre	Post	Pre	Post	Pre	Post
Average														

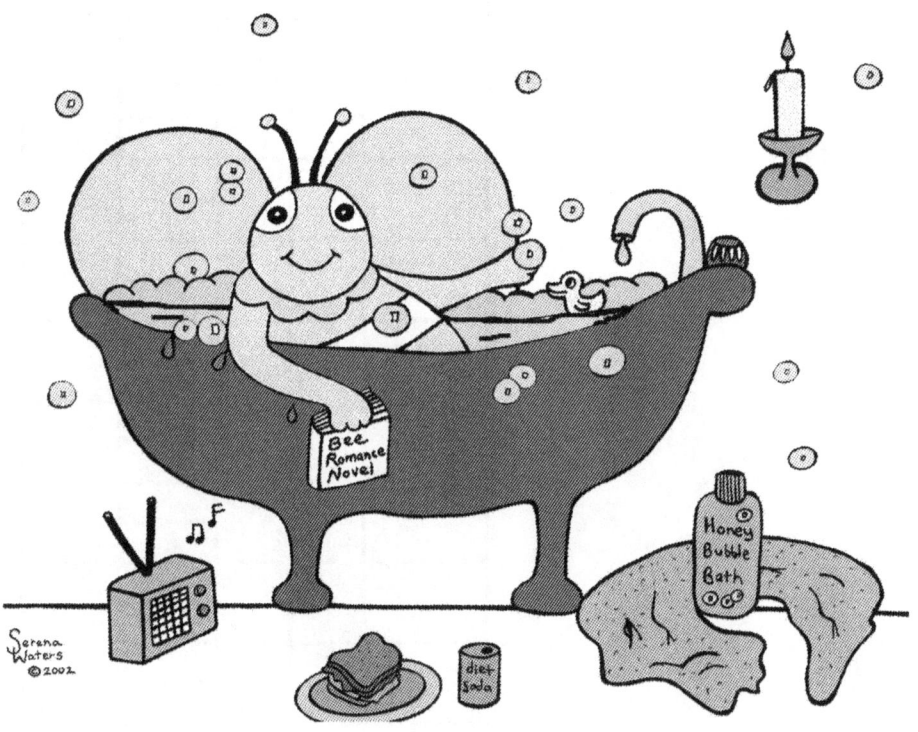

Treat yourself. Time for you is essential.

Time	Monday,_____ Meals and snacks	Carbs or Exchanges	Glucose Reading		Insulin	Meds
			Pre	Post		

Carbohydrates / Exchanges _____ Total _____ Goal

Journal your exercise, thoughts or feelings here.   Ketones _____

_____
_____
_____

Time	Tuesday,_____ Meals and snacks	Carbs or Exchanges	Glucose Reading		Insulin	Meds
			Pre	Post		

Carbohydrates / Exchanges _____ **Total** _____ **Goal**

Journal your exercise, thoughts or feelings here.   Ketones _____

_____
_____
_____

Time	Wednesday,_____ Meals and snacks	Carbs or Exchanges	Glucose Reading		Insulin	Meds
			Pre	Post		

Carbohydrates / Exchanges _____ **Total** _____ **Goal**

Journal your exercise, thoughts or feelings here.   Ketones _____

_____

_____

_____

Time	Thursday,_____ Meals and snacks	Carbs or Exchanges	Glucose Reading		Insulin	Meds
			Pre	Post		

Carbohydrates / Exchanges _____ Total _____ Goal

Journal your exercise, thoughts or feelings here.   Ketones _____

_____

_____

_____

Time	Friday,_____ Meals and snacks	Carbs or Exchanges	Glucose Reading		Insulin	Meds
			Pre	Post		
Carbohydrates / Exchanges _____ **Total** _____ **Goal**						

Journal your exercise, thoughts or feelings here.   Ketones _____

_____

_____

_____

Time	Saturday,_____ Meals and snacks	Carbs or Exchanges	Glucose Reading		Insulin	Meds
			Pre	Post		

Carbohydrates / Exchanges _____ **Total** _____ **Goal**

Journal your exercise, thoughts or feelings here.   Ketones _____

_____
_____
_____

Time	Sunday,_____ Meals and snacks	Carbs or Exchanges	Glucose Reading		Insulin	Meds
			Pre	Post		
Carbohydrates / Exchanges _____ **Total** _____ **Goal**						

Journal your exercise, thoughts or feelings here.   Ketones _____

_____

_____

_____

Week of _____

Blood Glucose Summary

Time	Mon		Tues		Wed		Thurs		Fri		Sat		Sun	
	Pre	Post	Pre	Post	Pre	Post	Pre	Post	Pre	Post	Pre	Post	Pre	Post
Average														

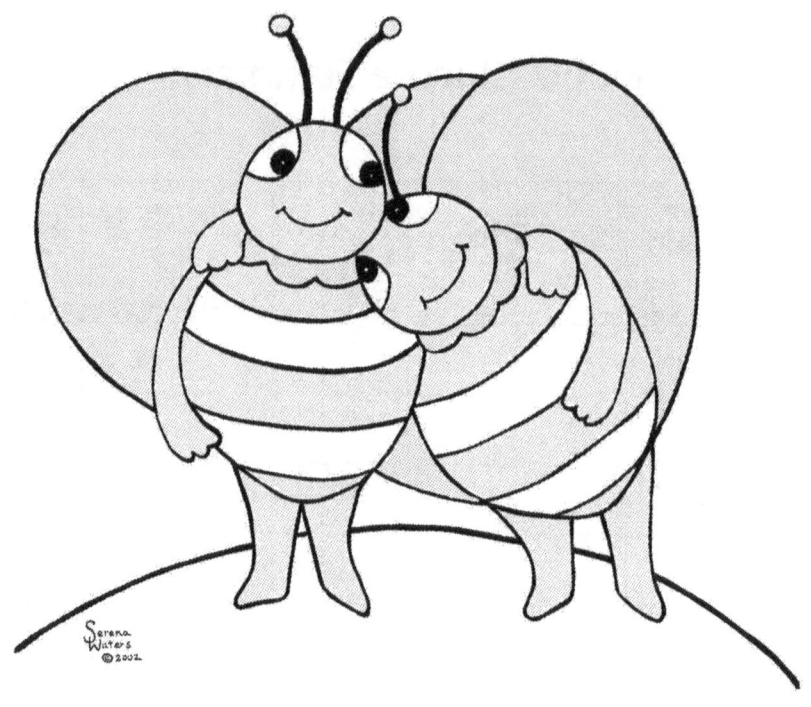

Bee a friend and support others who have diabetes.

Time	Monday,_____ Meals and snacks	Carbs or Exchanges	Glucose Reading		Insulin	Meds
			Pre	Post		

Carbohydrates / Exchanges _____ Total _____ Goal

Journal your exercise, thoughts or feelings here.   Ketones _____

_____
_____
_____

Time	Tuesday,_____ Meals and snacks	Carbs or Exchanges	Glucose Reading		Insulin	Meds
			Pre	Post		

Carbohydrates / Exchanges _____ Total _____ Goal

Journal your exercise, thoughts or feelings here.   Ketones _____

_____

_____

_____

Time	Wednesday,_____ Meals and snacks	Carbs or Exchanges	Glucose Reading Pre	Post	Insulin	Meds

Carbohydrates / Exchanges _____ Total _____ Goal

Journal your exercise, thoughts or feelings here.   Ketones _____

_____
_____
_____

Time	Thursday,_____ Meals and snacks	Carbs or Exchanges	Glucose Reading Pre	Post	Insulin	Meds

Carbohydrates / Exchanges _____ Total _____ Goal

Journal your exercise, thoughts or feelings here.　　　Ketones _____

_____

_____

_____

Time	Friday,_____ Meals and snacks	Carbs or Exchanges	Glucose Reading		Insulin	Meds
			Pre	Post		

Carbohydrates / Exchanges _____ Total _____ Goal

Journal your exercise, thoughts or feelings here.   Ketones _____

_____
_____
_____

Time	Saturday,_____ Meals and snacks	Carbs or Exchanges	Glucose Reading		Insulin	Meds
			Pre	Post		

Carbohydrates / Exchanges _____ **Total** _____ **Goal**

Journal your exercise, thoughts or feelings here.   Ketones _____

_____
_____
_____

Time	Sunday,_____ Meals and snacks	Carbs or Exchanges	Glucose Reading		Insulin	Meds
			Pre	Post		

Carbohydrates / Exchanges _____ Total _____ Goal

Journal your exercise, thoughts or feelings here.   Ketones _____

_____
_____
_____

Week of _____

Blood Glucose Summary

Time	Mon		Tues		Wed		Thurs		Fri		Sat		Sun	
	Pre	Post	Pre	Post	Pre	Post	Pre	Post	Pre	Post	Pre	Post	Pre	Post
Average														

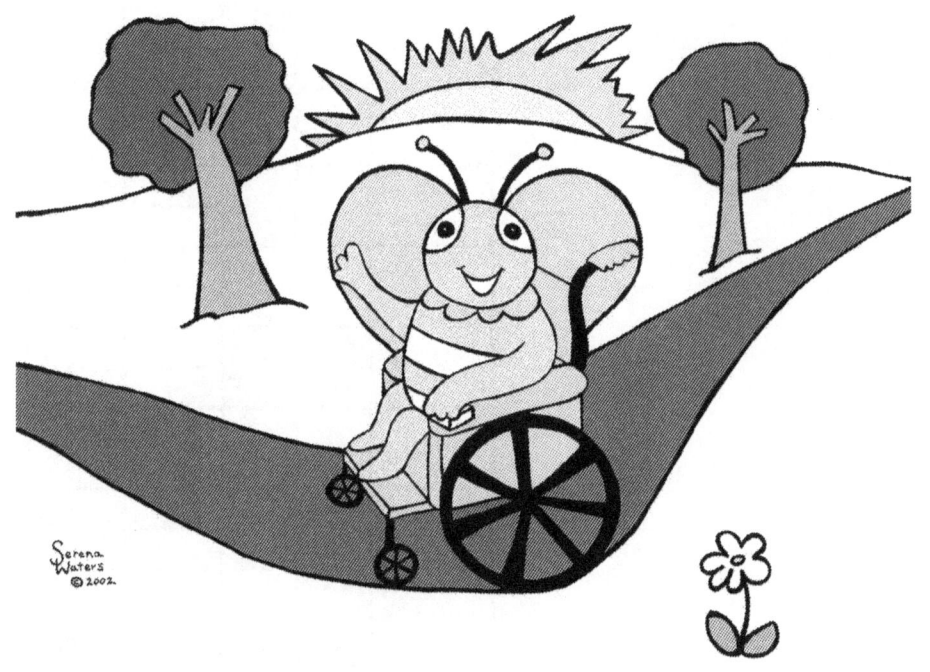

Keep rolling!
There may be bumps, but your dreams wait.

Time	**Monday,**_____ Meals and snacks	Carbs or Exchanges	Glucose Reading		Insulin	Meds
			Pre	Post		

Carbohydrates / Exchanges _____ **Total** _____ **Goal**

Journal your exercise, thoughts or feelings here.   Ketones _____

_____

_____

_____

Time	Tuesday,_____ Meals and snacks	Carbs or Exchanges	Glucose Reading		Insulin	Meds
			Pre	Post		
Carbohydrates / Exchanges _____ **Total** _____ **Goal**						

Journal your exercise, thoughts or feelings here.   Ketones _____

_____

_____

_____

Time	Wednesday,_____ Meals and snacks	Carbs or Exchanges	Glucose Reading		Insulin	Meds
			Pre	Post		

Carbohydrates / Exchanges _____ **Total** _____ **Goal**

Journal your exercise, thoughts or feelings here.   Ketones _____

_____

_____

_____

Time	Thursday,_____ Meals and snacks	Carbs or Exchanges	Glucose Reading		Insulin	Meds
			Pre	Post		
Carbohydrates / Exchanges _____ **Total** _____ **Goal**						

Journal your exercise, thoughts or feelings here.   Ketones _____

_____

_____

_____

Time	Friday,_____ Meals and snacks	Carbs or Exchanges	Glucose Reading		Insulin	Meds
			Pre	Post		

Carbohydrates / Exchanges _____ Total _____ Goal

Journal your exercise, thoughts or feelings here.   Ketones _____

_____
_____
_____

Time	Saturday,_____ Meals and snacks	Carbs or Exchanges	Glucose Reading		Insulin	Meds
			Pre	Post		

Carbohydrates / Exchanges _____ **Total** _____ **Goal**

Journal your exercise, thoughts or feelings here.   Ketones _____

_____
_____
_____

Time	Sunday,_____ Meals and snacks	Carbs or Exchanges	Glucose Reading		Insulin	Meds
			Pre	Post		

Carbohydrates / Exchanges _____ **Total** _____ **Goal**

Journal your exercise, thoughts or feelings here.   Ketones _____

_____

_____

_____

Week of _____

Blood Glucose Summary

Time	Mon		Tues		Wed		Thurs		Fri		Sat		Sun	
	Pre	Post	Pre	Post	Pre	Post	Pre	Post	Pre	Post	Pre	Post	Pre	Post
Average														

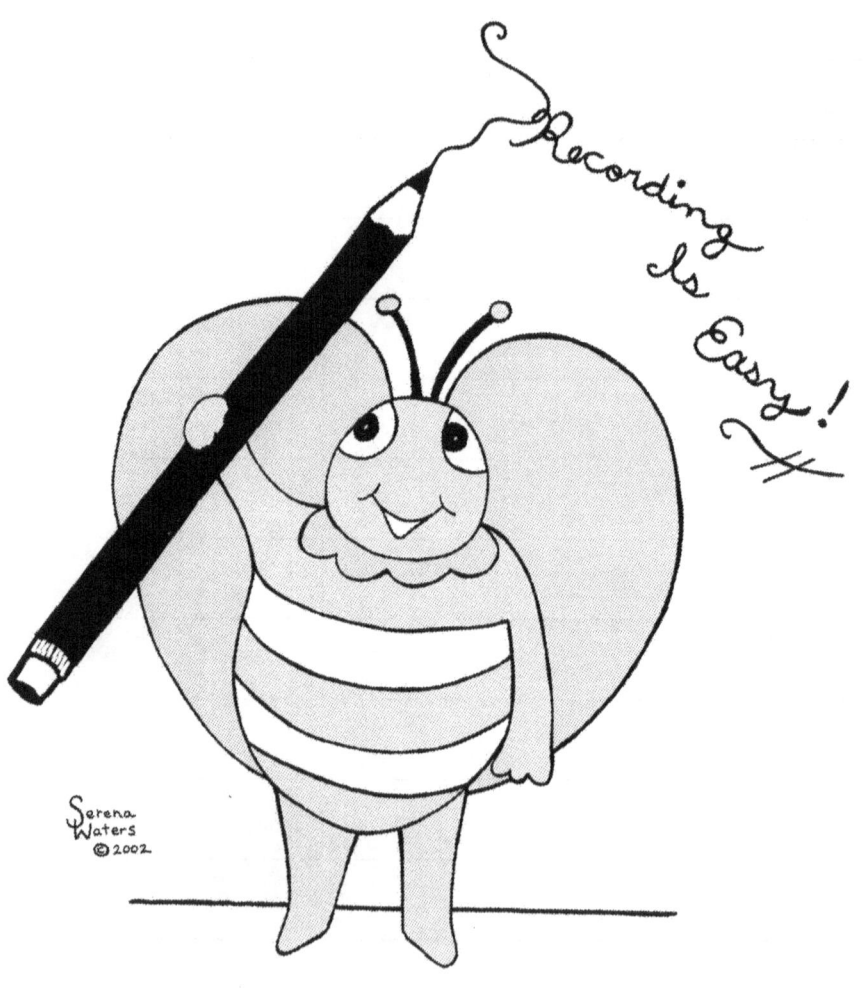

Time to reorder your "Bee Healthy Diabetic Log Book". Congratulations on a great six months!

For questions, comments or correspondence
please contact Sharon at: barker@albanytel.com

0-595-27117-0